TERESA SHIEI

SWEET FREEDOM
STUDY GUIDE

LOSING WEIGHT AND KEEPING IT OFF WITH GOD'S HELP

"If you stick with this, living out what I tell you, you are my disciples for sure. Then you will experience for yourselves the truth, and the truth will free you."

John 8:32 MSG

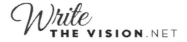

SWEET FREEDOM STUDY GUIDE
LOSING WEIGHT AND KEEPING IT OFF WITH GOD'S HELP

Printed in the USA

ISBN: 978-0-9910012-7-9 Print

Published by Write the Vision | Columbia, Missouri

Write THE VISION.NET

To Contact the Author:

www.TeresaShieldsParker.com

ACKNOWLEDGEMENTS

THANKS FOR BEING YOU!

I will be honest. This study guide was harder to write than I thought it would be. With the book done, I thought I could whip through it quickly and that my projected deadline would be no problem. That just wasn't true.

Sharing these concepts without sitting across the table from you, looking you in the eyes, asking questions and getting insights into what is going on inside you proved more difficult than I anticipated. However, when I would get stuck as to where to go next, God would pull me out and point me in the right direction. Together we finished this book for you.

My prayer now is that these principles become real to you and helpful on your journey.

As always I couldn't have gotten done without the help of a faithful team. Many thanks go to Shannon Fox, who gathered the initial data for this guide from *Sweet Freedom*. She pulled together the structure of the Chapter Lessons while I was working on the Principles. She is my right-hand gal on many of my writing projects. She'll outgrow me one day and then where will I be?

A special shout out goes to those who read, proofed and edited this study guide. These include my awesome team:

SWEET FREEDOM STUDY GUIDE

Shannon Fox, Marilyn Logan, Karen Fritzemeier, Michelle Smith, Rhonda Burrows, Mary Jennie Bodard, Linda Ordway and others. Thanks for your suggestions, positive comments and encouraging words.

Special thanks to Wendy K. Walters, as always, for the cover design. Her covers always "put the lipstick" on any book. And this is a book with some more explanatory content along with step-by-steps ideas for your study.

I could not have completed *Sweet Freedom* and *Sweet Freedom Study Guide* without the steady vigilance of the "watchmen on my wall".[1] The 23 faithful members of TSP Prayer Group prayed whenever I sent a request. Many prayed at special times for the book, for its contents, its title and for you, the readers. I will never undertake writing a book without a dedicated prayer team.

A special thanks goes to members of Sweet Change Weight Loss Coaching Group and #KickWeight coaching class. Whether or not you know it, you are my inspiration. You, and all those who want to be set free of food addictions, are why I keep doing what I do.

Special thanks to my family, Roy, Andrew, Jenny and her husband, Nigel, for putting up with me through this hibernation project better known as writing a book.

Above all, thanks to God Almighty who reminds me daily it was for freedom that I was set free.

ENDNOTES

1. Isaiah 62:6 NLT

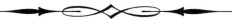

D E D I C A T I O N

*To all those caught in the literal
hell of food addiction.*

*To all those who want to do what is
good, but don't. Who don't want to do
what is wrong, but do it anyway.*

To all those who know what to do

*and seriously have a desire to
transform completely,*

*but find themselves stuck in
the same endless loop.*

*Finally, there are answers and
you will find them here.*

I wrote this book for you.

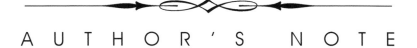

FROM MY JOURNAL

"Fix your attention on God. You'll be changed from the inside out."

Romans 12:2 MSG

There is no better way to begin to teach a lesson than to share with you a glimpse of how I communicate with God and He with me. There are many other ways, of course. I am led daily by Him, as you are. This teaching time I'm sharing to begin this journal is an important foundation for this journey we are taking together.

MY QUESTION:

Lord, before anything else I want You and You alone. How do I communicate with others that if they do not make You their number one they fail in a major way? This goes way beyond the body thing of weight gain. It's about their very lives. It's about where they will spend eternity. It's about the abundance (or lack thereof) that they will enjoy (or miss) while here on earth.[1]

GOD'S ANSWER:

Tell them I am.[2] I am the one who made them and I know all about them. I know their weaknesses and their tendencies. I fashioned grace so they don't have to rely on things that seem close and at hand. Those things are but substitutes for Me. They may seem like tremendous substitutes, but they don't hold a candle to Me and My grace.

Grace wasn't just a thought or invention of Mine. Grace is who I am. People need to understand that my justice is grace, just as my forgiveness is grace. Without a means to judge a person, grace is not needed. Those who are far away from Me and miss the mark, as every person has, deserve punishment.[3] That's justice. The remedy for that is grace through the Person of Jesus. He is grace personified because He and I are One.

You, My creation, make grace so difficult and yet, it is so simple. Because sin entered the world, the human condition requires sacrifice. Jesus is and was that sacrifice.[4] No one, no matter how good, can keep every law in the book. It's not possible. Break one law and you are guilty of breaking them all. And everyone has broken at least one law. Who among you has never lied? There isn't one of you, I know. I see everything.

Grace for Living

That's another thing, you think I don't see you eating things that are harmful for you. It makes me extremely sad because you are damaging your body, the house where I have lived[5] from the moment you accepted Jesus' sacrifice. I have great and awesome plans for you. You do have a future. Disaster for your life is not My plan.[6] But if you damage your body there will be disastrous results for you.

I do heal. I do restore. What good does it do for Me to heal and restore you if you don't follow the principles of taking care of yourself? If you are running to earthly things to comfort and sustain you rather than to Me, you are not following all that I have for you. I want you to be in good health. I want you to be healthy in body, soul and spirit.[7]

There are reasons why I say You should worship Me and Me only should you serve.[8] Nothing else. I don't care what it is. It may be a really good thing, oh, like church or chocolate pie, but if you are putting them first instead of Me, you are in disobedience!

Grace for Worship

Dear Children, I love you with an everlasting love. I am drawing you to Myself with arms of grace, strength and love. Come to me. Rely on Me. Do You think My arm is too short[9] to draw you close and embrace you in the light of My presence?

Have you ever really felt my presence in a real and tangible way? Ask for Me to come and I will. I will come and I will touch. I will heal. I will restore the years[10] when you have cooperated with the enemy to destroy your very being.

Grace for Failure

Give Me all your shame, all your regret, all your guilt. You do not have to carry it any more. I will take it if you will release it. Give it to Me right now. Then ask Me, "What do You give me in return?"

I will give you good gifts that will be far and above anything you have ever in your wildest imagination dreamed. I will promote you. I will fight for you. I will be your God in a way you have never seen before.[11]

You are burdened with the cares of this world so much that you cannot see your hand in front of your face. Look up! Yes, I am the lifter of your head,[12] but right now you must activate and look full into My eyes of love.

You first have to make a move towards Me. Until you do, you effectively tie My hands, but when you move, repent and fall before Me, I will run to meet you.

Grace for Restoration

The father of the prodigal son did not try to go find him. It would have been a fruitless effort. He allowed him to come to the end of his resources.

Only then did the son make the decision to turn from what he was doing and return home. When the father saw him, He ran to him and welcomed him with a hug bigger than any he'd ever been given.[13]

In that moment it all began—restoration, healing and release to live in abundance.[14] It all began when the son, by returning home, admitted his failures and wrongs, and the father, by his solid welcome home, extended the magnanimous grace of heaven.

TO THE READER

What does God require of you today? He simply requires that you start towards Him. The principles in this study guide can help. However you must put your whole body, soul and spirit into understanding God is waiting for you to begin. Lift your head. Look full in His face. He's waiting for you to take the first step. He promises to meet you there. You have to initiate the process. Then, you must join Him in running towards His heart for you.

I warn you, though, this is not some idle commitment. This is a full out run. This is an I-do-this-with-everything-within-me abandonment. This is I-stop-everything-else-and-focus-on-You agreement between you and the God of the universe.

FIRST ACTION STEP

Get a clean spiral binder or journal. Use this to write your response to discussion questions, insights in your Bible reading, notes as you go through activities. Make this your *Sweet Freedom Study Guide* notebook. Decorate it. Personalize it. Carry it with you to meetings or to work. Write insights at lunch or break. Don't let it out of your sight.

First question to answer. Where is my commitment level to this journey and why? Is it where I want it to be? What must I do to get it to where I know it needs to be?

Write out your commitment to God. Dear God, I commit to... Now, whatever happens, if you find a group or are in a group, if you find an accountability partner or not, you are committed to this journey. There's a reason this page should be your first page in your journal.

NEXT

There are two parts of this study guide. The Principles section includes an overview of the inner healing processes mentioned in *Sweet Freedom*. The Chapter Lessons follow that. That begins with "How to Use the Chapter Lessons". At the end is a Next Steps section. The Principles section also comes with Action Steps.

The Chapter Lessons have various activities, discussion and thought-provoking questions, Bible study questions and suggested music for each session.

Because the Chapter Lessons use the Principles, they are first in this guide so you can familiarize yourself with them. You could just study the Principles, but then you'd miss the awesome activities and questions. Nope. Better do it all!

ENDNOTES

1. John 10:10 NLT
2. Exodus 3:14 NIV
3. Romans 3:23, 6:23 NIV
4. Romans 5:20-21 NIV
5. 1 Corinthians 6:19 TLB
6. Jeremiah 29:11, NLT
7. 3 John 2, 1 Thess. 5:23 NIV
8. Luke 4:8 NIV
9. Isaiah 59:1 NIV
10. Isaiah 38:16 NASB
11. Ezekiel 36:28, Exodus 14:14 NIV
12. Psalm 3:3 KJV
13. Luke 15:20, NASB
14. John 10:10 NASB

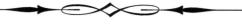

C O N T E N T S

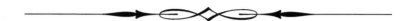

"So here's what I want you to do, God helping you: Take your everyday, ordinary life—your sleeping, eating, going-to-work, and walking-around life—and place it before God as an offering. Embracing what God does for you is the best thing you can do for him. Don't become so well-adjusted to your culture that you fit into it without even thinking. Instead, fix your attention on God. You'll be changed from the inside out. Readily recognize what he wants from you, and quickly respond to it. Unlike the culture around you, always dragging you down to its level of immaturity, God brings the best out of you, develops well-formed maturity in you."

Romans 12:1-2 MSG

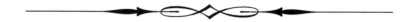

PRINCIPLES

FORGIVING OTHERS

E ver since I can remember, I've wanted to get along with everyone. If I knew someone had something against me, I would go to the person, talk it through and try to come up with a solution. I tried not to step on toes. I wasn't forgiving them, however. I was trying to negotiate a settlement where we both could win. I was trying, in some way, to get them to agree with me.

When I was 60 years old, I grew up. Throwing yourself in the public limelight will make you realize you are never going to please everyone all the time. People will disagree with you and that's OK. They are entitled to their opinion. If you're breathing and talk at all, you will make someone angry at some point in time.

Before I came of age, it would have devastated me that someone would disagree or even be angry with my point of view. Today, I am OK with divergent points of view as long as people do not try to force me to agree. If they do, I simply walk in forgiveness. If they speak or write angry words, it's not worth holding on to any pain they cause. It doesn't hurt the other person if I am angry. As a matter of fact, it only damages me. Jesus says it actually puts us in prison when we don't forgive things others do to us.[1]

HOW TO FORGIVE

How do I forgive a random person who says bad things about me, cuts me off in traffic or makes a rude gesture? Do I hunt them down and tell them I forgive them for doing that? What if they don't want to be forgiven? Can I still be mad at them then?

Forgiveness is an attitude of my heart. I don't have to say it directly to them. It doesn't matter if they want to be forgiven or not. I am setting myself free from their negative influence over me when I choose to forgive them. Forgiveness simply means acknowledging to God, "I choose to forgive that person for what they said or did."

FORGIVING OTHERS SETS ME FREE

These simple words meant from the heart will set me free. I choose to forgive them and let their words or actions go. As a matter of fact, I send their words back to them. I take back any of my self-respect, courage or energy they stole from me, washed through the blood of the Lamb. By sending their words back, I don't mean I repeat what they said. I mentally send those words back to the source. It's now theirs to deal with. I forget it and move on.

If they are still angry and volatile, it is their issue. I've learned some people will simply choose to be angry. They do not feel alive unless they are angry about something. I do not have to allow them to continue speaking into my life. I do not have to allow their words to ruin me. I do not have to also be angry because they are. I simply choose to not allow whatever happened to affect me.

FORGIVING THOSE WE LOVE OR HAVE LOVED

It can be more difficult to forgive someone we love or have loved who has damaged us in some way. Maybe it's an ex-spouse or former significant other. Maybe it's a relative. Maybe it's a close friend. Maybe it's a boss, pastor or church board member. When they betray, manipulate, abuse, lie, cheat or cause any other harm to us, our first response is to harbor the hurt and play the victim.

When we refuse to forgive, we add years to our hurt and pain. The harm they did may take only a few minutes or months to inflict upon us, but we extend it by decades when we don't forgive. They have moved on with their lives and have most likely forgotten what they did or said, but we are stuck with how we feel.

Forgiving them and handing them to God releases us to live again. We may forgive them once and expect the hurt to be gone. The key to remember is forgiveness is a process. We do it until it is done.

We simply say, "I choose to forgive this person for what they have done. I send the hurt they did to me back to them. I take

5

back what they retained of me, my innocence, courage, trust (or other harm done) washed through the blood of the Lamb."

When feelings or thoughts of that person return to our minds, we take those thoughts captive to the obedience of Christ.[2] We don't dwell or wallow in the hurts and difficulties of the past. We simply go through the process and state again, "I choose to forgive..."

TURN THE CHANNEL

Then, we intentionally think about something else. We count our blessings. We meditate on Scripture. We turn on praise music. We sing and dance to the music. We read a good book, go for a walk, hug a child, feel the breeze on our skin and rejoice that we are alive to experience the day. We turn the channel of our mind.

If we allow ourselves to meditate on the situation, we open the door to depression. In depression or to stave off depression, we often go to artificial substances, such as alcohol, drugs or food to alleviate the harbored hurts. We need to get busy, find something productive to do, pray and read the Word or journal our thoughts. We may need to get medical, psychological and spiritual help. Most of all, though, we need to forgive.

When we feel someone has hurt us, we will worry the situation to death. I remember a former pastor explaining it like this: "Worry is praying to yourself." When I worry over a situation it usually means I am not able to fix it and make it turn out like I want. When I tear apart a circumstance from every angle and try to put it back together, all I am doing is worrying and trying to manipulate people to be who I want them to be. It is a my-will-be-done situation.

The truth is, I cannot fix what happened. I can't make someone be nicer, stop controlling me, get a job, stop doing drugs, stop overeating or be a better parent, spouse, child or friend. I have to let God deal with that person. I should be careful to not enable their poor choices. All I can control is me and my reactions. This also means I may have to choose to no longer be in a close relationship with them until they make some changes.

Many situations feel impossible. What we can do is pray for the person, hand them to Jesus and not grab them back out of His hands. We can share God's truth when the person wants and is ready to hear it. I've found short memorable Scriptures or statements dropped in conversation at the right time can be life-changing. God may use us or someone else to get individuals we love to a place of forward movement.

WE CANNOT FORCE CHANGE ON OTHERS

One thing I constantly keep in front of me when coaching another is I can't want change for the person I'm coaching more than they want it for themselves. They must want to change. I can't force it on them. If I do, they will recognize that and rebel. I must forgive and put them back safely in the arms of God.

"There is no one like the God of Israel. He rides across the heavens to help you, across the skies in majestic splendor. The eternal God is your refuge, and His everlasting arms are under you. He drives out the enemy before you."[3] This is the power of the God we serve. Why we ever think we have the power to fix our loved ones without His help is beyond me.

I've heard people say, "They don't deserve to be forgiven for what they did." I always want to answer, "Did you deserve for God to forgive you?" No one deserves forgiveness. However, God sees you and me as much of a sinner as the person who wronged us.

For us to not forgive another, no matter what they have done, would be like God refusing to forgive us for our shortcomings. God commands us to forgive because it sets us free from carrying hatred, bitterness and anger with us for the rest of our days. We have to trust Him on this.

Remember, if you don't forgive them, it puts you in prison, not them. Like I've heard Joyce Meyer say, "Unforgiveness is like drinking poison and expecting the other person to die." Holding on to hurts can actually cause me to have health issues. So if I want to stop feeling so crummy all the time, I need to try forgiving the deep things which have been causing me pain.

GOD'S COMMAND

God commands me to forgive others. He says if I don't forgive others, He won't forgive me.[4] He also tells me before I pray I am first to forgive anyone I am holding a grudge against so God will forgive me.[5] This says to me if my prayers don't seem to be getting through, I should check my attitude towards others first.

Forgiveness is a humongous deal to God. Since it is so important to Him, it should be to me as well. Remember the story of the unforgiving debtor? It comes right after Peter asks Jesus, "How often should I forgive someone who sins against me? Seven times?" And Jesus replied, "No not seven times, but seventy times seven." [6]

THE UNFORGIVING DEBTOR

Jesus doesn't stop there. He tells a story.[7] The Kingdom of Heaven can be compared to a king or master who decides to settle accounts with those who owed him money. One man owed the master millions of dollars and couldn't pay anything. So the master ordered that the man and his family be sold into slavery.

The man appeared to humble himself and begged the master to let him pay it off. Instead the master went one step further and forgave all the debt.

What did the man do in response? He went out and found a man who owed him a small amount in comparison to what he had owed the master and demanded instant payment. That man begged for mercy, but the unforgiving debtor had him arrested until he could pay it.

"Then the angry king sent the man to prison to be tortured until he had paid his entire debt. That's what My heavenly Father will do to you if you refuse to forgive your brothers and sisters from your heart."[8]

I don't know about you, but I don't want to be in prison. In real life, if a person goes to a prison he is still his father's child. The problem is in prison he is not free to do as he wishes. He finds himself confined, restrained, stuck. He longs for his old freedoms.

Spiritually speaking, Jesus came to set us free. Our job is to make sure we stay free.[9] One way we can put ourselves in bondage is to hold on to offenses and refuse to forgive.

Christ died to set us free. When we ask for forgiveness He gives it freely. He expects His children to follow His example. Since we have been forgiven we are to forgive others. It's that grace thing again.

I have no idea why God didn't have me sign a contract when I accepted Jesus as my Savior. The contract should have said, "Teresa will never eat candy or sugar again." He knew my tendencies. He knew what would happen when I didn't listen to His advice about how to keep my body, His house, in a way that it honors Him.[10] Yet He gave me grace for the sins I had already committed and the many more I would commit.

IS EATING SUGAR A SIN?

Is eating sugar a sin? For me it became a sin the minute I asked Him how to lose weight and He told me to stop eating sugar. Whenever I refuse to follow His instructions I sin, whether the instructions come through prayer or His Word. Of course, eating sugar is only the tip of the iceberg of ways I've failed God.

The point is we have all sinned,[11] and yet He gives us His grace when we accept His Son as our Savior. "Through the blood of His Son, we are set free from our sins. God forgives our failures because of His overflowing kindness. He poured out His kindness by giving us every kind of wisdom and insight."[12]

We are forgiven in order that we might show the grace of God to others and forgive as well. Will it be easy? I think it's a whole lot easier than spending life in prison, but I'm not willing to find out.

ACTION STEP

What about you? Who do you need to forgive and for what? Open your journal. Label a page "Forgive Others" and make three columns. Name them "Who," "What" and "When". Under "Who" write the names of people who have harmed you in some way. It can be small or large hurts. It doesn't matter if you've forgiven them or not.

Under "What" write what they did. You may have numerous entries for each person. That's all right.

Under "When" write when you chose to forgive them if they are forgiven. If you don't remember when, just write the general timeframe such as childhood, young adult, adult, last year, just some way for you to see the timeframe.

The ones you have not yet forgiven are open loops in your life causing harm to yourself in some way. When you are ready, go through and forgive those individuals by simply stating, "I choose to forgive (the person) for (what they did)." Write the date.

Make it your goal to choose to forgive the others on the list. Begin to pray about any reasons you can't or won't forgive them. Ask God to teach you more about forgiveness and its importance in your life.

Think about how great you'll feel when you can say you have no areas of unforgiveness or open loops in your life.

Each day make it a habit to pray like Jesus did in the Lords' prayer.[13] "Forgive me today for what I've done wrong against You, just as I forgive others who have wronged me. Show me if there is someone I need to forgive today."

ENDNOTES

1. Matt. 18:24-25 NLT
2. 2 Corinthians 10:5 NIV
3. Deuteronomy 33:26-27 NLT
4. Matthew 6:14-15 NLT
5. Mark 11:25 NLT
6. Matthew 18:21-22 NLT
7. Matthew 18:23-33 NLT
8. Matthew 18:34-35 NLT
9. Galatians 5:1 NLT
10. 1 Corinthians 6:19-20 NLT
11. Romans 3:23 NIV
12. Ephesians 1:7-8 GW
13. Matthew 6:12 NLT

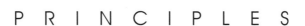

THE GOD CONNECTION

W̲e are a spirit. We are a soul. We are a body. These three parts make up who we are. Because we are human, each part of us has needs. These needs are basic to who we are. What would it look like if we created a picture of ourselves, our needs and those who have provided those needs and where we should get those needs today?

Pictures always communicate the truths of God best to me. So let's look a picture like that only in the form of a chart which might help us to remember it better.[1]

This chart is based on the fact that God Himself sees as a tri-part being—body, soul and spirit.

"May God Himself, the God of peace, sanctify you through and through. May your whole spirit, soul and body be kept blameless at the coming of our Lord Jesus Christ. The One who calls you is faithful, and He will do it."[2]

I call this The Connection because to me that's what it is. It shows clearly in what areas the part of God we know of as the

Trinity, relates to us. Of course we know God is beyond our comprehension and not limited to what He has revealed to us of Himself.

I suggest you recreate this chart in your journal. Open your journal and turn it sideways. On the top write, The God Connection. Divide the horizontal page in three columns and label them, Family, Me and My Needs and Godhead. Divide the page into three rows. You should have nine blocks on your page. Under the Family label each block, going down the rows vertically, first, Dad or father figure, then in the next block,

THE GOD CONNECTION

FAMILY	ME AND MY NEEDS	GODHEAD
Dad or Father Figures	**Body** Identity or Self-worth Protection Provision	Father God
Siblings, Peers or Close Friends	**Soul** Companionship Communication	Jesus
Mom or Mother Figures	**Spirit** Comfort Teaching	Holy Spirit

Siblings, Peers or Close Friends, and the next, Mom or mother figure. Under God label each block going down the rows vertically, Father God, then Jesus, and in the next block Holy Spirit.

In the middle column under Me and My Needs, there will be several things to write. In the first block going down write, Body, and under that in the same block list one under each other, Identity/Self-Worth, Protection, Provision. As you read horizontally across the page you should have Dad or father figure and in the next block, Body, then the other three things I just told you to write. In the last column, Father God.

Going down vertically under Body write, Soul, in the next block. Then under Soul list Companionship, Communication. Going down vertically to the last block, the one under Soul write, Spirit, and then list, Comfort, Teaching.

You will refer back to this chart as you go through inner healing. We'll also add scriptures, especially in the needs area. The chart shows body needs are identity and a sense of self-worth, protection and provision. Soul needs companionship and communication. Spirit needs comfort and teaching. It also shows the roles of our family and the members of the Godhead in relationship to our needs.

UNDERSTANDING

I like to add Scriptural understanding to any method I use for inner healing. The Scriptures clearly show three persons of the Trinity relate to each part of us—body, soul and spirit.

God is ultimately responsible for these areas in our lives, however our families should give us a clear picture of this.

Many times, due to circumstances or other issues, our perception is they do not take care of our needs. This short-circuits our view of who God is and how He can provide for us completely in each of these areas.

You may have a lot of knowledge about Scripture. You may have been taught the principles of who God is. You may have even taught them yourself. The truth is, if you know the principle, but still don't feel you can trust God to provide one or more of your needs, you have an emotional disconnect with Him.

Where does this emotional dissonance come from? It probably stems back to something which happened in your childhood.

SCRIPTURES

Before discussing that further, let's examine the Scriptures. There are examples of each of these categories throughout the Bible. I challenge you to do your own search and find the verses which speak the loudest to you in each of these areas. Here are some places to begin. List these in the appropriate places on your chart.

Identity and Self-Worth

"Oh Lord, You have examined my heart and know everything about me...You go before me and follow me. You place Your hand of blessing on my head," Psalm 139:1,5 NLT.

Protection

"You are my hiding place; You will protect me from trouble and surround me with songs of deliverance,"[4] Psalm 32:7 NIV.

Provision

"Your heavenly Father already knows all your needs. Seek the Kingdom of God above all else, and live righteously, and He will give you everything you need," Matthew 6:32-33 NLT.

Companionship

"And it came about that while they were conversing and discussing, Jesus Himself approached, and began traveling with them," Luke 24:15 NASB.

Communication

"And they said to one another, 'Were not our hearts burning within us while He was speaking to us on the road, while He was explaining the Scriptures to us?" Luke 24:31 NASB.

Comfort

"But when the Comforter is come, whom I will send unto you from the Father, even the Spirit of truth, which proceedeth from the Father, He shall testify of me," John 15:26 KJV.

Teaching

"But when the Father sends the Advocate as my representative— that is, the Holy Spirit—He will teach you everything and will remind you of everything I have told you," John 14:26 NLT.

FAMILY

If perfectly constructed, our family has three parts, father, mother and siblings. Our earthly father is the one tasked with providing the needs and wants of our body, our mother with those of our spirit and our siblings, peers or friends with that of our soul. [3]

As we are growing up we may perceive our needs weren't met in some area. I've found this can be in obvious or hidden ways. When our needs don't get met we get wounded.

If our father was absent for a legitimate reason, such as work, we may feel we were not protected and are fearful. If our mother was sick, worked long hours, traveled a lot or had too much to do to pay attention to us we may perceive we weren't comforted.

If our siblings, peers or other relatives our age manipulated us or ridiculed us we may feel ashamed.

These perceptions take place in childhood during a time we cannot cognitively process them. So, not knowing how to handle them, we bury those feelings. Unfortunately they still govern how we feel even into adulthood if we don't take care of them.

GODHEAD

If we don't process any disconnect with our family members it will effect how we feel about the members of the Godhead who have the same roles.[4] If I perceive my earthly father or father figure didn't protect me, then I may feel Father God can't or won't protect me. I may have solid knowledge of the Scriptures and may be able to quote the words, but emotionally I feel unprotected.

It will likely cause me to be fearful. If I perceive my earthly mother didn't comfort me, I may find alternative comforts in addictive behaviors, food being a major one. The problem here is I know the Holy Spirit is the Comforter, but instead I go to something I can see, touch, smell and taste because I think I need comfort I can control. I have no paradigm for the Holy Spirit comforting me because all I got from my mother or mother figure was food.

If I perceive my siblings or peers ridiculed me, I may feel I cannot have a relationship with Jesus. I can't talk to Him because He might do the same thing. Jesus, though, is the One who lived as a human, like me. He is the member of the Godhead who is meant to walk and talk with me as my best friend.

RECONNECTING

Disconnects can happen in any area. Any time we feel a disconnect with God in some way it probably goes back to some emotion we have buried deeply because of a misperception, hurt, wounding or situation in our childhood.

Some of these may have come from loving and caring people who didn't realize the effect their words or actions have had on us. Many people have problems forgiving a mother, father, grandparent or sibling they love and who feel didn't do anything wrong.

They didn't intentionally do something wrong, however to you, the little kid, at the time it felt wrong. That child inside you wants his or her feelings to be recognized. In some ways, they are still governing your emotions even though you have become an adult. The process of forgiveness through to hearing God's truth will set you free in profound ways.

The person you are choosing to forgive may already be in heaven, but your feelings are still here on earth with you. You are not pointing fingers and telling them or the world they were bad. You are simply releasing tons of emotional baggage connected to the child inside you who was in some way damaged through faulty perceptions.

Some damage may have come from selfish individuals who were out only for themselves, not caring at all about us. In both cases, the key to getting a solid connection with God is forgiving individuals we perceive have harmed us. This is not the type of forgiveness where you go and confront the individual. It is not necessary for reconnection to God unless God reveals to you that you should do this.

In *Sweet Freedom* I share many various ways I have approached this. There are basically two ways: picturing God and working with a presenting issue.

PICTURING GOD

If I told you to put a picture of an elephant in your mind, you could do that easily, right? Picturing God is the same thing. It is not using some kind of guided imagery, it is simply another method of understanding if you have a solid connection with Him.

Put a picture of Jesus, Holy Spirit or Father God in your mind. This is how you see this member of the Godhead, not how you are supposed to feel or see Him. Whatever you see, hear or sense first would be what you want to pay attention to.

Where is He? Is He close or far away? How large or small is He compared to you? Where are you? What does it look like? What colors are present? What do you sense? What do you feel?

Your picture of Father God will reveal how you feel about Him. It will also reveal some of your relationship with your earthly father and how that relationship impacted you in various ways. Same with Holy Spirit and mother or Jesus and siblings. An example of this in the book is in the chapter called "Control" where I saw my painting of Jesus.

After seeing your picture ask that member of the Godhead, "Is there a lie I am believing about You? What is the lie?" When you understand the lie, ask Him, "What is the truth?"[5]

If you have a great relationship with everyone in your family, but God reveals a disconnect, don't be afraid of going through this process. God is revealing a hidden area of lies the little child in you believes.

Going through this process will only bring you closer to that individual. It will not push you further apart. He will reveal truth to you through this process. Finally, "you will experience for yourselves the truth, and the truth will free you."[6]

Action Step: Find a quiet place and time. Do this with each member of the Godhead. Take notes. You may want to note what lies He told you and especially what His truth is.

PRESENTING ISSUE

God may reveal to you areas which need to be healed. A certain issue may arise such as not being able to trust God to be with you during certain aspects or times in your life. Many times my issues don't seem to relate to the place I end up. In the chapter titled "Unprotected", I was afraid God would no longer help me on my weight loss journey.

What I do when I sense there is an issue in my life, I ask the member of the Godhead I think would relate to that, "When is the first time I felt this fear?"

It is necessary to go to the earliest incident. When we go to the root, which is always in childhood, then we can cut off the issue through forgiveness.

Allow God to help you remember the issue and the person who was the root source of your feeling. Notice the person who is making you feel whatever you felt.

In this instance for me it was my dad who relates to Father God. (Refer to the God Connection Chart.) I forgave Dad, renounced the lie Father God would treat me the same way and asked Father God what His truth was.

My grandmother was also involved. You can go back to the chapter to see how I forgave her. This still seemed to be a Father God issue because Grandma also felt fear. In this situation I gave Father God the anxiety I felt from Grandma. In exchange He gave me peace. More about exchanges later.

PAINFUL TIMES

Many times presenting issues are painful. We don't like to remember something which hurt us. That's the reason we bury them. Sometimes, though, they can rule our lives.

An example of this is in the chapter "Fear". The incident with Fred[7] at the time seemed monumental in my life. He loomed like a monster I could not overcome. Forgiveness was the real key to overcoming this issue.

Getting to the root of this is similar to the presenting issue. Presenting issues can also be painful memories.

This approach, though, begins with remembering the incident, understanding which member of the Godhead relates and then going through the process. This may lead you to another painful memory, like it did for me with Adam.[8]

THE GOD CONNECTION PROCESS

By now you should have an understanding of whom to forgive and which member of the Godhead relates to that situation. Here is a summary of the steps you need to go through, filling in the appropriate information. Find a quiet place and time when you can be alone. Say the following out loud to God. Repeat what He says back to you.

(Father God, Jesus or Holy Spirit) I choose to forgive (person, usually father, mother, sibling or friend) for (the specific perceptions you have and specific circumstance where those began).

I renounce the lie You, (Father God, Holy Spirit or Jesus depending on the person you forgave) will (make me feel or will do the same things you forgave the person for in #1).

Now, (Father God, Holy Spirit or Jesus) what is Your truth? You have just asked the God of the universe to tell you a truth. He will answer you. Don't overthink this. We have done that all our lives. Note the first thing you see, hear or feel. Write it down. If you don't understand it, ask Him to show you. Don't rationalize. Just accept His answer. Write it down.

(Father God, Holy Spirit or Jesus) what do you think of me? Write down the first thing which crosses your mind. Spend some time seeing if what you heard matches God's Word. Write down the Scriptures He shows you.

Action Step: Find a quiet place and time. Ask God if there is some issue you need to deal with. If you don't know where to start, you might begin with the needs column. Ask Father God, "Am I afraid?" If He says, "Yes," ask, "When is the first time I felt afraid?" Or you might know what the issue is. If so say, "I feel afraid. When is the first time I felt this or what is the root of the fear?" Then, go through The God Connection process.

Here are a few other questions and the probable member of the Godhead they relate to. I say probable because as you read *Sweet Freedom* you'll understand I've been surprised many times by His answers. So see it as a place to begin on the journey. Choose one from the list or your own and begin this amazing journey!

Jesus

I feel like I have no friends.

How can a Spirit-being be my best friend?

Do You even know me?

How can I get out of this mess?

Do I trust You?

Can I talk to You?

Why do I feel like food is my best friend?

Why do I feel so alone?

Father God

Will you make sure we have enough money to pay the bills?

Are you really willing to take care of me and my family?

Why do I feel like I don't know who I am?

Why do I feel like I'm headed nowhere when I have a great job?

Why do I feel like I am a nobody in the kingdom?

Do I have a destiny and if so how can I get there?

Why am I so afraid when I know You say You will take care of me?

Why do I think I have to protect myself?

Holy Spirit

Why am I so sad and depressed?

Why do I feel anxious?

Why am I so mad about everything?

Why do I need food, alcohol, drugs, cigarettes, pornography, shopping, gambling or other things to comfort me when I know it is harmful for me?

How do I face tomorrow?

How can I get this task done?

Why does it feel like I'm swimming through mud and I can't do this any more?

Remember, you can ask God any question. To me it always seems as if He's sitting on the edge of His throne waiting to lead me to the answer.

ENDNOTES

1. "Tools." Sozo Basic Manual. Redding: Sozo Ministry, 2011. 31. Print.
2. 1 Thessalonians 5:23-24 NIV
3. "Tools." Sozo Basic Manual. Redding: Sozo Ministry, 2011. 31. Print
4. "Tools." Sozo Basic Manual. Redding: Sozo Ministry, 2011. 34. Print
5. "Tools." Sozo Basic Manual. Redding: Sozo Ministry, 2011. 36-37. Print.
6. John 8:32 MSG
7. Not his real name
8. Not his real name

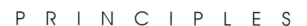

BARRIERS

H ave you ever said, "It just seems like I've hit a wall in my relationship with God"? Or how about this, "It feels like my prayers are just bouncing off the ceiling. It's like I can't get beyond that barrier."

When it is difficult to hear from God or a certain member of the Trinity, there may be a barrier or wall we have knowingly or unknowingly erected to serve as a form of protection from others or even God.

Many times these barriers will also be built by us in order to keep a member of the Godhead out of the situation. Or we may have put them up to protect ourselves from memories which are too traumatizing for us to remember.

It's good to ask God before trying to dismantle any wall, "Is it safe for me to remove this wall?" Barriers we put up to protect ourselves in childhood may have been God's way of keeping us safe then. We may still need it to feel safe or it may be time to ask God to help you dismantle it. Always ask first.

When going through the God Connection exercise and you just can't see, hear or sense anything, there is probably a wall or barrier. Don't worry, though, once the wall is gone, reconnection with God is the best reward.

REMOVING A WALL OR BARRIER

Ask whichever member of the Godhead you can talk to the best and ask, "Is there a wall or barrier in my life?" Ask, "Will You show me the wall?" Close your eyes and picture it.

Be open to anything you see, sense or hear. It may be a void, a color, an object or an actual wall. Notice what it is constructed of, the color, where you are, what is on your side of the wall, what you can see, hear or sense is on the other side. Note your feelings as you picture the wall.

Ask Him, "Is it safe for the wall to come down?" If the memories are too much to take all at once, God may tell you it's not safe for the wall to come down.

If He says, "Yes," then ask Him, "How can this wall be moved? Will you give me a tool to remove it?" God may give you something which seems odd to use to remove the wall.

If you have no sense of how to use it, ask God, "How do I use this tool to remove the wall?" If it seems too difficult, ask Him, "Will You help me remove the wall?"

Picture the wall being removed or you using the tool to remove it. When the wall is gone, picture what or who is on the other side.

If, for instance, Father God was helping you remove the wall and on the other side you see Jesus. If the wall is down, you can now run to Jesus. You may want to invite Father God to come with you and then, also invite the Holy Spirit.

I share a couple of instances of this in *Sweet Freedom*. One is the tangled briar wall with snakes in the "Fear" chapter. There is also the donut wall, the chocolate tomb and the nothing wall. If you only see a color that can also indicate a wall. Simply ask the Holy Spirit, your teacher, what it means if you don't know.

Again, this is why I call all of these principles The God Connection. It has seriously changed my prayer life. I now am asking Him teach me more about who I am and how to exchange the lies I believe for His truth. I'm also honestly seeking His face, not His hand. I want to know who He is.

BETTER RELATIONSHIP

Removing a wall is always designed to facilitate a better relationship with the entire Godhead. Remember each Person of the Trinity has specific roles which are necessary for you to become a whole person. Your goal is to be able to embrace and feel comfortable with the totality of God that is knowable.

We can never know all of God. He has dimensions we can't fathom. He is infinite. I am finite. Yet, this infinite being chooses to dwell and make His home in me, a flawed human being.

I want to know Him intimately. It is something I seek. However, I cannot ever really arrive there. In this life, I can only be on the journey with that as my destination.

It is in the midst of the mystery of all that God is that I joyfully live.

ENDNOTES

1. "Tools." Sozo Basic Manual. Redding: Sozo Ministry, 2011. 45. Print.
2. Ibid.

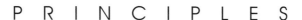

EXCHANGES

An exchange is simply handing God something you no longer wish to carry and asking Him, "What do You give me in exchange?" It's not demanding He give you something, but it is understanding what He gives you in exchange will be something very valuable to you on your journey.

Exchanges are all throughout the Bible when you open your eyes to see them. He gives us new life for our old one.[1] He gives us the possible for our impossible.[2] He gives us beauty for ashes, joy for mourning and the garment of praise for the spirit of heaviness.[3] When we give Him our shame, He gives us double honor. We give Him our disgrace, He gives us rejoicing in our portion and everlasting joy. [4]

We give Him our poverty of spirit. He gives us the kingdom of heaven. We give Him our mourning. He gives us comfort. We give Him our meekness. He gives us an inheritance as big as the earth.[5]

We give Him hunger and thirst for righteousness. He fills us. We give Him a merciful attitude. He shows us mercy. We give Him pureness of heart. He gives us Himself.[5]

We give Him our weakness. He gives us His power. We give Him our insults, hardships, persecutions and difficulties. He gives us His strength to keep going.[6]

We give Him what we feel is holding us back, no matter what that is. He gives us exactly what we need to move the next step forward.

It's a simple process. It is not heart-wrenching, foaming at the mouth or writhing on the floor like some see deliverance. It is simply handing to God what seems overwhelming in our lives, and like the good Father He is, He gives us the tools we need to go forward on our journey.

ACTION STEP

Make a list of all the things you feel are holding you back such as fear, anger, constant hunger, rebellion, loneliness, shame, greed and anything else. Then, one at a time, take each thing symbolically place it in your hands, close your eyes and say, "Father God, I give you fear. What do you give me in exchange?"

As with other tools we have talked about, whatever you sense, see or hear Him speak to you in your mind will be what He gives you. Write down each gift He gives you next to the thing you gave Him. Then, ask Him to show you how to exercise His gift to you.

Do the same thing with people in your life with whom you are having issues. It could be a relative or friend who is wayward. Someone who is too dependent on you or you on them. Someone who has a disease or injury. As you hand them to Him and ask what He gives you in exchange, picture that person safely taken care of by the God of the universe.

You will undoubtedly want to repeat this process again and again. Writing down what you give Him, and what He gives you in exchange is a great way to remember that promise from Him.

Find Scriptures which help you understand more about His gift to you. Ask Him to teach you how that gift will help you go forward.

ENDNOTES

1. 2 Corinthians 5:17 NLT
2. Matthew 19:26 NIV
3. Isaiah 61:3 NKJV
4. Isaiah 61:7 NKJV
5. Matthew 5:3-8 NIV
6. 2 Corinthians 12:9-10 NIV

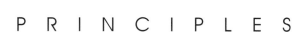

DOORS

There are said to be four doors. This theory was developed by Pablo Botari, a pastor from Argentina. He believes all strongholds or issues stem from the opening of these four doors.[1]

I've found most people I've had the privilege of coaching through this process understand and relate primarily with the door of fear. However, there are also the doors of hatred, sexual sin and witchcraft.

These are symbolic doors inside you. There are many reasons why these doors could be open in your life, but all will stem back to some incident, probably in your childhood.

I've found that once I understood this process, the evil one loves to hide issues behind doors where they don't seem to belong. I talk about that in the chapter called, "Control". Don't be frightened by that. Just check each door to see if it is open or closed and if it is open, investigate the potential reasons why it might be open.

With witchcraft, which seems to be a tricky one, ask God, "Will you reveal to me any point in time where I might have opened this door?" Pay attention to what crosses your mind after you ask that. The deceiver will try to live up to his name.

DOOR OF FEAR

It feels like Satan loves to keep this door open. As a child we can be fearful about many things. We are little. The world and all the people in it are humongous.

Fear can cause us to do many things. We self-protect and comfort ourselves with harmful life patterns such as indulging in drugs, alcohol, sugar or many other addictions.

We worry about things which are out of our control and, therefore, try to control everything. We are anxious because of our lack of control which makes us want to isolate ourselves from anything and anyone who can harm us.

Unbelief and apathy also tend to keep this door open. If we don't believe and don't care maybe fear will leave us alone.

I used to live here. I'm so glad today I live in the place that grace built! (See the Sweet Freedom chapter, "The Place That Grace Built".)

DOOR OF HATRED

The door of hatred can have many things that trigger that door being open. Self-hatred is the most common one among those I deal with. That negative self-worth can cause that door to be left open until we deal with the root.

My postulation is that all the other things that may indicate the door is open stem from self-hatred. We just don't love ourselves like Jesus tells us to do in the Great Commandment.

"Love the Lord your God with all your heart, soul, and mind. This is the first and greatest commandment. The second most important is similar: Love your neighbor as much as you love yourself."[2]

We can't love our neighbor if we don't love ourselves. We will be doing the other things which open the door of hatred. We will gossip, envy, be bitter, slander and be angry with others.

Finding out who or what is keeping the door of hatred open is the first step to making sure that door is tightly shut and sealed by the blood of the Lamb.

The principle of the door is mainly to check with yourself to see if there is any area which hasn't been taken care of in your life. It is simply a tool to give you an idea of what might be hindering you in your life.

Here are the basics for seeing if there is a door open. I would only use this if you have tried every other resource and still have no idea what is holding you back. It is also a good place to begin the connection process because it can reveal to you where to start on your journey.

DOOR OF OCCULT/WITCHCRAFT

Satan likes to rule various domains and this is one he likes to revel in. Many times we think we surely don't have an open door like this in our lives. However, Satan rarely comes to us dressed in bright red footie pajamas with a hood and horns carrying a pitchfork. We should check this door to see if there is anything which could have remotely entered through this door when we weren't watchful.

Many times this does happen in childhood. Innocent toying with astrology, fortune telling, tarot cards, seances, Ouija board can open the door. Just doing one of these things does not mean the door is open unless it has left the door of intrigue into that realm open.

If so, that can lead to the deeper things of witchcraft practices, casting curses and participation in covens. An interesting part of this is what I call a manipulative spirit. This is also lurking behind this door.

Christians can definitely have a manipulative spirit hiding behind a mask of Christianity. It appears in the form of "follow me as I follow Christ."[3] It is only manipulation when certain people or cults try to do this to garner money, time or resources from other people. In other words to benefit themselves or their organization. It takes a discerning spirit to recognize this in others and be open to examine in our own lives.

Where a manipulative spirit exists, there may either be a door of witchcraft open or they may simply not know they are influencing others totally for their own benefit.

DOOR OF SEXUAL SIN

This is a critical door to examine in our lives because many things in today's culture can open this door, especially if we keep gazing at and longing for what lies beyond that open door. Pornography is a big one here. Many enter this door through the gate of television, the internet, magazines and even romance novels.

Pornography itself can be very addictive. For Christians it appears as a way to provide pleasure without "sinning". However, as has been proven by the testimony of death row prisoners, pornography can lead to rape, molestation and violent crimes.

It is also a gateway to adultery and fornication, basic unfaithfulness. Which, of course, leads to the rise in the divorce rate and rising lack of commitment to marry in the first place.

DEALING WITH OPEN DOORS

Now that I've taken you through this list of doors, what do we do if we find a door open in our lives? This process is really a checkup to tell whether or not there are any presenting issues left to deal with.

If there is an open door, ask the member of the Godhead you are most comfortable with who or what is holding the door open or you may know instantly who or what is holding it open. Go through the God Connection Process again, forgiving the person who is holding the door open. Or trace what is holding it open back to a specific incident and begin The God Connection Process there.

Finish the process with renouncing the lies, hearing God's truth and reconnecting in a real way with Him.

It may lead to an exchange or tearing down a barrier. Whatever happens, the great thing about open doors is they can be shut. Bringing a member of the Godhead in to nail the door shut, seal it with the blood of the Lamb or secure it in a fashion that gives you comfort that it will remain closed is a good way to make sure it stays closed.

ACTION STEP

Close your eyes and picture the door of fear. Is it open or closed? Open may mean it is open for fear to enter your life or come and go as it pleases. If it is wide open, it may mean you are extremely open to fear or even taken over by fear. If it is closed solidly, locked and bolted, it can mean fear is absent.

Go through the God Connection process to deal with who or what is keeping the door open. Then, come back to that door and see if it is closed. If not, forgive, renounce and hear truth again.

As a coach said to me when I was complaining about having to forgive my mother for what seemed like the zillioneth time, "Forgiveness is a process. We do it until it is done."

I say a closed door "can" mean fear is not present because I have known people who felt they were locked inside of fear, hatred, sexual sin or witchcraft and could not get out.

If this is the case, ask the member of the Godhead you are most familiar with, "Who has locked me in here or have I locked myself in here?" Ask, "Who am I afraid of?"

When you understand those answers, go through The God Connection process again, forgiving, renouncing lies and hearing God's truth. It is always a great relief to close and seal a door shut, knowing the God of the universe Himself is going to stand guard there for you.

ENDNOTES

1. "Tools." Sozo Basic Manual. Redding: Sozo Ministry, 2011. 39. Print.
2. Matthew 22:37-38 NLT
3. 1 Corinthians 11:1 MEV

CHAPTER
LESSONS

HOW TO USE
LESSON GUIDES

BEFORE THE STUDY

Do the action step in the Author's Note "From My Journal". Be sure to write your name in the journal you create so if it's lost you can find it. Keep this with you or have a way to take notes and transfer them to the journal when you get home. Jot the notes on your phone or anywhere. Once you get started on this journey, God will begin speaking to you at odd times.

You should have a copy of the *Sweet Freedom: Losing Weight and Keeping It Off* and the *Sweet Freedom Study Guide*.

BIBLE VERSIONS

Sweet Freedom uses several versions of the Bible in this study, most of these are available free online at Biblegateway.com. *The Passion Translation* is a new translation, which is not yet out in the complete Bible. The ones in *Sweet Freedom* are *John: Eternal*

Love; Proverbs, Wisdom from Above and *Letters from Heaven by the Apostle Paul*. All Scriptures referenced, whether from *The Passion Translation* or other versions of the Bible will be printed out in this study guide. However, if you wish to purchase for your own devotions, you can find them on Amazon.com.

PRAYER PARTNER

If doing the study alone, consider asking someone to be your partner to study together. If no one wants to join you for the study, ask someone to be your prayer and accountability partner.

ESPECIALLY FOR LEADERS: GROUP RULES

Read the rules during your first session. You may want to read these for the first few sessions or remind your group of them if new people come in.

• **Confidential:** Keep everything said in the group as confidential. Weight issues and addictions are very personal. Individuals may have never before shared what they will share in your group.

• **Honest:** Sharing should be real and honest. No embellishing. No lying. No half-truth.

• **Open:** Being open and transparent about your issues is the first step to healing. This is a place where you can share your junk, and in doing so, begin to release it.

• **Safe:** Stress to your group this is to be a safe place. Share only your stuff, not what the lady on your block did. Do not share in large group what your partner shared unless she or he asks you to. That is theirs to share and it is part of being confidential even within the group. Own your stuff and share that.

- **Emotional:** It's OK to share your emotions—cry, laugh and even express dissatisfaction. We do not have to stuff our emotions in this group. Be loving and accepting of every person no matter where they are on their journey.

USING THE LESSON GUIDES

Leaders, feel free to use what parts of each Lesson Guide work best for your group, size, facility and time constraints. There are many questions in each section. Use any or all of them at your discretion. There is also an activity for each chapter. In many cases this can also be used to facilitate discussion. Do not feel you must do everything in each chapter. Encourage your group to study the lesson on their own and then come ready to discuss and learn from each other. Make sure everyone knows what unit to study for the next session.

COMMITMENT

It goes without saying there should be commitment to this study. Read or review the *Sweet Freedom* chapter for the week, read the lesson guide and think about or answer the questions. Be faithful to come unless providentially hindered, which doesn't mean your favorite movie is on.

Leaders, encourage members to contact them to let them know if they are not able to come. Make sure everyone knows how best to contact you.

STARTING TIME AND SETUP

Whatever the announced starting time, keep to it. It goes without saying that as the leader you need to be on time or early. You should have an assistant leader who is available if you are running late. Don't set the example of being late, then members will be late. Still, there may be those who come in late.

Do not repeat everything for latecomers. This only reinforces the behavior of those who are always tardy. As a leader, be there early and have the room set up like you want.

Your group size will determine room set up. A circular format tends to work best if the group is not too large and your room is large enough for the circle. Some sessions may work better at tables. Plan according to what is scheduled for the session. Announce when you will be there and encourage group members to come early for fellowship.

MATERIALS

You may wish to have name tags and a roster with check in and any session handouts at a table where individuals enter. Vary the way they do nametags. Ask them to draw a symbol with their name. One session maybe the weather you love, an animal that symbolizes you, the last thing you ate, where you'd like to go on your next vacation, a fruit you like or a vegetable that signifies you. After the group has gotten to know each other, ask them to sign it as a Bible character they identify with. Be creative.

Review each session at least a month in advance. Certain sessions will require additional materials. Many of these are items people have at home like fabric scraps, items from nature, old magazines, markers, nail polish, dress up materials, etc. Planning is key.

Asking members to bring materials they have at home will take the burden off the leader. Don't count on them to bring it the day of the meeting. Have them bring the items in advance so you know you have everything you need to make the session a success. Note one of the first sessions for the Author's Note and Introduction has construction paper and items to use for a collage.

MUSIC

Music is great to open each session with. If you have a phone or mp3 player with music downloaded, you can use that with an inexpensive Bluetooth speaker to play a song to begin or end your study. Many are suggested with each session. Feel free to substitute ones that work best for you and your group.

If you are studying on your own, set the tone of your study time with one of the suggested songs. Most can be found on YouTube. If lyrics aren't included, it's great to look them up and print them out for those in your group or even for yourself.

As a leader, it's great to put others in charge of different aspects. Be sure whoever is leading is not afraid of standing in front of people and singing along with the music. Worship, have fun, praise God to begin your study!

PRAYER

Near the beginning have an opening prayer to invite the presence of the Holy Spirit into your study. There will be some deep things discussed. You want His total leadership and anointing on the meeting. Here's simple, but powerful prayer to start your meeting. "Holy Spirit, Come. Lead us. Guide us. Teach us."

There is a prayer section in each unit. Prayer is a key, however, let's make the prayer personal. It's good to pray for all kinds of needs, but for this study let's focus on what action steps we need to take, and what we feel God is asking us to do. This is a perfect way to end your session. Let partners pray together and allow them to pray and leave when they finish.

GROUPS AND PARTNERS

This study guide and individual lessons are designed for you to use for personal or group study. It would easy for a small or large group to complete. In all cases it is helpful to have partners for accountability and sharing.

To begin the study let members choose partners. Then, in a few weeks encourage them to get with someone they don't know well. In a few more weeks, invite them to pair up with someone they haven't partnered with before. Be creative. One-on-one time is great for building new relationships.

FIRST SESSION

Leaders, it's always your decision where to begin and how to lead your group. There are several ways to start. "Begin at the Beginning" is a lesson that is not connected to any chapter in *Sweet Freedom*. It is designed to make sure everyone is on the same page spiritually. It is also a time to get to know each other and where everyone is on their faith journey. However, if you already know everyone in the group you may want to just encourage the members to read this lesson.

The lesson guide for the Author's Note and Introduction can go together with the beginning lesson. The lesson guide for this has mainly questions to think about. You may want your group to simply study these two sessions on their own and then start your study with the chapter "Listen".

Wherever you begin, go over the rules for the group and set the tone in the first session. You may use any portion of the material in any session. There will be notes to leaders for suggestions, but please be led by the Holy Spirit and don't feel you have to cover all the material in each session. Give assignments so the group knows what will be covered in the next session.

The "Begin at the Beginning" session is a good place to start because participants do not have to have read the book or the study guide to come to that session. From there you can give assignments.

As a leader, when you have partner time or small groups, walk around and enter into discussions. Especially note if groups or partners are not talking. Casually enter in to get them started.

CONNECT WITH TERESA

If you begin a group in your church, please let our team know by emailing info@TeresaShieldsParker.com. You may use this email for any questions or if you would like to invite Teresa to speak at your church or event.

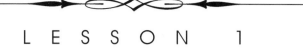

BEGIN AT THE BEGINNING

Note: This lesson is not related to a chapter in Sweet Freedom. However, it is material necessary for each member to understand and embrace to really go on this emotional and spiritual journey. An option is to assign this chapter and perhaps the next related to the Author's Note and Introduction as something each can study on their own.

Song: "All This Time" by Britt Nicole.

Read: Read Teresa's testimony. What is your testimony?

Is there a time when you have accepted Christ as your savior? Has there been a time you feel you have walked away from Him or not done what He has told you to do?

Do you feel you are doing what He wants in the aspect of how you eat, how you move and whether or not you are emotionally healthy?

What are some areas that need more work?

TERESA'S TESTIMONY

I accepted Jesus as my Savior when I was seven. That is, I said the words, walked the aisle at church, prayed the prayer, and after that I felt I had the ticket to heaven. Just to be sure I lived what I considered a good Christian life, went to church every week and did what the preacher said to do. I was religious.

There was always a constant striving though to do more, be more, earn my way into God's good graces. I was soon to learn that grace had nothing to do with what I did and everything to do with what God did for me.

When I realized I was a sinner (Romans 3:23) and was bound for hell if I didn't accept Christ as my savior (John 3:16), it was a no brainer for me as a kid. I accepted Him in order to stay out of hell.

In doing that, I got grace. Because of grace, God set me free from trying in any way, shape or form to earn salvation. How could I earn what I already had?

When I became an adult, my eyes were opened to the fact I was really living in disobedience to Him. I rejected what He told me to do back in 1977. I kept eating sugar and tons of starches. I didn't begin focusing on meats, fruits and vegetables. I wanted to eat what I wanted. I wanted my comfort foods.

I began trying to do more "works" for Him to make up for my disobedience. Surely more good deeds would outweigh what I was reserving just for me.

My true repentance moment came when I understood I was addicted to sugar. I surrendered what had been standing between God and me. I laid it on the altar, turned around and went the other way.

I've often wondered when the real point of salvation was for me. Was it at age seven when I had the initial understanding or at age 55 when I surrendered the thing I loved more than even God?

When we come to Christ, we are made new. The old is gone and the new has come. How new could I have been made when I was seven? At that point on my journey I didn't know much. I learned later some of what I accepted as truth was not God's truth, but mine.

God didn't give up on my misbeliefs and faulty thinking. He continued to work with me until I clearly began to tap into the higher level of understanding of God's power.

SURRENDERING MY FIRST LOVE

What would have happened to me if I had never surrendered my first love, which was clearly comfort food? To be honest, I'm not sure. I wasn't all the way new in terms of how 2 Corinthians 5:17 puts it. Still, I was in the process of being made new.

I know I am still in that process. I believe we all are. It doesn't matter to me now whether I was saved when I was seven or 55. There is no doubt in my mind now. I am His, sold-out 100 percent.

In my foodie years, I would repent and pray the salvation prayer again during every church service. It would last about as long as it took to get to the restaurant for lunch.

I don't know the real answer to when I was actually "saved". I just know now that I am now. I did fully accept Christ back in 1960, at least with as much faith as a seven-year old can. I think I lived the faith of a seven-year old for years. Jesus says we have to come with the faith of a child. However, He means for us to grow and continually get closer to Him in our faith.

I also know the doubt and wondering was driving me crazy. Why do I continue to disobey Him if I am saved? If this is where you are now, don't stay in doubt. Get it settled now.

READ AND WRITE

Read the following Scriptures. Stop and write in your journal about any Scripture or portion of Scripture that arrests you, stops you or makes you think. Ask, "Jesus what are you saying to me?" Write what you think He's telling you. Please note, the evil one will try to distract you during this time. Don't let him. Especially do not allow his lies to creep in during this time. Focus only on what you know to be right. You have asked Jesus, the Son of God, to communicate with you. Allow Him and Him alone to speak into your life.

Romans 3:23 NLT—"For everyone has sinned; we all fall short of God's glorious standard."

Romans 6:23 NLT— "For the wages of sin is death, but the free gift of God is eternal life through Christ Jesus our Lord."

John 3:16 NLT—"For this is how God loved the world: He gave His one and only Son, so that everyone who believes in Him will not perish, but have eternal life."

Ephesians 2:8-9 TPT—"For it was only through this wonderful grace that we believed in Him. Nothing we did could ever earn this salvation, not even our faith, for it was the gracious gift from God that brought us to Christ. So no one will ever be able to boast, for salvation is never a reward for good works or human striving,"

2 Cor. 5:17 NLT—"Anyone who belongs to Christ has become a new person. The old life is gone; a new life has begun!"

PRAY

Pray the prayer below or your own prayer. Pour out your heart to Jesus. You can know today, beyond a shadow of a doubt, you are His. Journal your prayer, sign and date it.

"Jesus, I need you to make me a completely new person. I want the old life to be gone. I want your new life. I surrender the things I have placed higher than you. I want you and you only. I accept you into my life. Show me the path I should walk and lead me into a deeper understanding of who you are."

SHARE

If you are doing this study alone, share what happened in this session with a friend or your pastor.

Leaders, depending on your group size, take time to get acquainted. Sharing where you are on this journey will be a great way to do that. Include anything, which stood out during this study.

If you are in a large group, divide into small groups to share. Set a time limit appropriate for all to share. One to two minutes will be enough. Give someone the responsibility of signaling time so the person talking realizes they need to wrap up. Some may monopolize the time if a limit is not set. Be cognizant of those who are shy and don't wish to share. Allow people to share when they feel comfortable.

If you are doing this study alone, share what happened in this session with a friend or your pastor.

SING AND CLOSE

Song: Play "I Believe (The Creed)" by Hillsong Worship.

Leader should close in prayer. Pray thanking God for who He is. Use the following or your own prayer.

"Thank You, Heavenly Father, for Your gift of grace. Thank You, Jesus, for loving me enough to die for me. Thank You, Holy Spirit, for making my body Your home. I love You, my God and my King. In Jesus' name, Amen."

AUTHOR'S NOTE INTRODUCTION

AUTHOR'S NOTE

Read the Author's Note in the beginning of *Sweet Freedom: Losing Weight and Keeping It Off With God's Help*.

In your notebook write and finish the following statements.

1. God, I admit my weakness for …..

2. If I could come away from this study with one thing, it would be ….

3. I commit to finishing this study and doing the work because ….

4. I am a….

5. I want to be …

Spend some time in the large group, in small groups or in two's sharing some of your answers. If you share with a partner, include some sharing time in the large group.

INTRODUCTION: BARRIERS

After reading "Introduction: Barriers" in *Sweet Freedom* take a moment to write your answers to the following questions:

1.   What are you struggling to overcome right now?

2.   In what way have your emotions held you back?

3.   What specific emotions scream at you the loudest? List these.

4.   How have you tried to overcome this struggle so far?

Again, spend some time in larger group, small group or in twos sharing some of your answers.

CREATE AND ACT

Ask God, "What barriers are keeping me from overcoming my personal struggle?" Be specific regarding which struggle you are referring to.

In your journal, write what you sense God said to you.

On a piece of construction or heavy paper, make a collage of what your barrier looks like. Use materials such as scraps of fabric, sticks, leaves, feathers, rocks, magazines, copies of favorite photographs or any other things you or those in the group can gather. You could also simply draw this.

Ask God, "What would sweet freedom look like for me?"

Make a second collage or drawing reminding you of what you sense sweet freedom looks like for you.

Share your collages and what they mean to you with a partner, small or large group.

PRAY AND SING

Pray this prayer out loud to remove the barriers in your life. (Refer to "Barriers" in the Principles Section.)

Leaders: Pray first out loud and invite the members to repeat after you.

"Father God, Thank You for being here and teaching me tonight. Right now I thank You for showing me the barriers which I have erected in my life for protection. I thank You that You are my Protector. Now, Father God, show me the wall I have erected."

(Pause for God to work on hearts and minds and to listen to what He is saying to you.)

"I simply ask You, if it is safe, will You remove this wall right now?"

(Pause and give time for God to work. Then, ask, "Is the wall removed?" If not, ask the members to pray the following.)

"Father God, can You give me a tool to remove, tear down or obliterate this wall? And will You show me how to use the tool and together can we remove this wall?"

(Pause again. Then, ask all to repeat after you.)

"Thank you, Father God, that you want sweet freedom for me more than I want it for myself. Show me what that looks like for me. In Jesus' name, I pray."

Song: Play "Thank You, Jesus " by Hillsong Worship.

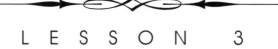

L E S S O N   3

LISTEN

THINK ABOUT IT

Have you sensed, felt or heard God speaking to you? If so, when?

How do you know it is God's voice and not someone or something else?

What is the last thing you know for sure God asked you or showed you that you did?

What is the last thing He showed you to do that you didn't do?

Do you trust God's voice to lead you?

READ AND WRITE

John 10:27 NLT—"My sheep listen to my voice; I know them, and they follow me."

Are you one of His sheep? Does He know you? In what ways do you follow Him? When is following Him difficult for you?

If you don't follow Him, what does that say about your relationship with Him? Are you still His sheep?

Hebrews 6:19-20 NIV—"We have this hope as an anchor for the soul, firm and secure. It enters the inner sanctuary behind the curtain."

How is God's voice like an anchor for your soul? (For more information read Hebrews 6:13-20)

Galatians 5:16-18 NIV—"So I say, walk by the Spirit, and you will not gratify the desires of the flesh. For the flesh desires what is contrary to the Spirit, and the Spirit what is contrary to the flesh. They are in conflict with each other, so that you are not to do whatever you want."

What desires are you following? List these. Are they leading you towards life or death? In what ways?

James 3:17 NIV—"But the wisdom that comes from heaven is first of all pure; then peace-loving, considerate, submissive, full of mercy and good fruit, impartial and sincere."

When is a time you remember this to be true? How have you seen this in your own life?

CREATE AND ACT

Think of a time when you were faced with making a decision. It could be a seemingly small decision like the one Teresa faced in this chapter. Label a blank page in your notebook something to remind you about that decision, such as Cinnamon Roll or Buying the TV.

Make three columns under the heading. Label them Tempter's Voice, My Voice and God's Voice. Beginning with the Tempter's Voice, list the things the Tempter would tell you about that situation. Under your voice, list what you might be saying to yourself. Note: The things you say to yourself may come from your mother, father, siblings or significant people in your life, as well as from yourself.

Now, list the things God would say to you and how you know it is Him. Use the list in this chapter in *Sweet Freedom* titled, "Ten Things I've Learned About God's Voice" to help you.

Think about a decision situation and go through the following exercise. If doing personal study, do this on your own.

Leaders: Ask for a volunteer from the group to share a decision situation. Do this activity as a group. Make sure you have a flip chart, white board or chalk board to write down the ideas from the group.

Ask the group, "What are some examples of ways we can make sure we are listening to the right voice?" Write these on the board and encourage the members to write them in their notebook.

Have members choose a partner in the group for them to be mutually accountable to or, if doing this on your own, ask someone to help you stay accountable. Covenant to pray together and help each you listen to God's voice, rather your own voice or the voice of the enemy.

Share specific situations where you have difficulty doing this. Get each other's phone number and text each other if a situation or temptation arises where you are having difficulty hearing

God's voice. Check up on each other with an encouraging text or call that says something like, "How's it going?"

SHARE, SING AND PRAY

Are you ready to have God's voice guide you with His wisdomrather than your own or the lies of the tempter? Are you ready to be led to a place of life, rather than a place of death?

Psalm 25:5 NIV—"Guide me in Your truth and teach me for You are God my Savior, and my hope is in You all day long."

Pray this prayer to God especially in regard to helping you hear God's voice in times of temptation and difficulty.

Song: Play the song, "Holy Spirit, Come and Fill This Place" by CeCe Winans. Ask the group members to invite the Holy Spirit to fill their hearts and make it His place.

Pray: Have one person pray for those in the group to hear from God, reject the tempter's voice as well as their own and give God permission to intervene in their lives.

"Dear Heavenly Father, Guide us with Your wisdom and truth. We want to hear Your voice above the noises in our heads and the tempter's voice. Speak clearly, God. Remind me when I'm going the wrong direction or headed towards difficulty. God, I give You permission to intervene in my life. I am seeking to dismiss the other voices, even my own, to hear ONLY Your voice. Teach me more of who You are, how You work in my life and the lives of others and what Your ways look like for me. We are Your humble servants. Thank You for leading us in Your paths of righteousness. In Jesus' name, Amen."

HOPELESS

SING

Song: "The Sound That Saved Us All" by Anthony Skinner.

THINK ABOUT IT

Ask the participants to think about how grace has been amazing in their lives. Ask one or two to share with the group. In your personal study, write down your answer.

When is a time you've thought or said, "I can't do that?" Is this really true?

What lies do you believe about this situation?

What is God's truth about it?

What opportunities have you denied yourself because of lies you believed?

How has God tried to get your attention? Did you listen? Why or why not?

READ AND WRITE

2 Corinthians 12:9 MSG—"My grace is enough. It's all you need. My power comes into its own in your weakness".

Is God powerful all the time? If so, then why is His power only activated when we admit our weakness?

Why are grace and power both involved in this Scripture? What does grace have to do with power?

Matthew 17:20 NLT—"You don't have enough faith," Jesus told them. "I tell you the truth, if you had faith even as small as a mustard seed, you could say to this mountain, 'Move from here to there,' and it would move. Nothing would be impossible."

Is there a time frame in this Scripture for mountain moving? Does it say it's going to be done in an instant? Do you believe God is big enough to move your mountain even if it takes a while?

How could mountain-moving look different than you have imagined it in the past?

What might you have to do in order to see the mountain move?

CREATE AND ACT

Role Play how you would handle various situations, which require God to move a mountain? Divide into groups of six or fewer. Leaders, instruct each group to choose one or more situations from the list below to discuss.

What would honestly be your first reaction in the situation you chose? What would you want God to do? What if He didn't do that? How would you react? What might be some reasons why God would not do exactly what you want? What would be the right way to handle this situation?

SITUATIONS

• You suspect your husband of 10 years is cheating on you. You have two small children.

• Your doctor tells you that you have five years to live unless you lose 100 pounds and keep it off.

• Your son just told you he is gay and is moving in with his partner.

• Your husband, who is a pastor of a large church, told you he has been embezzling hundreds of thousands of dollars from the church. The church doesn't know about it.

• You are diagnosed with stage 4 cancer. Doctors say you might have six months to live. You are single and have no children.

• You have $50,000 in credit card debt and your husband just had his hours cut at work.

After five minutes, have a spokesperson from each group share with the large group. If you have a small group, discuss as many situations as you have time for. If doing this study alone, write out your response in each situation.

Ask: How have you seen God move mountains? How long did it take?

PRAY

Dialogue: Ask God, "Why do I feel hopeless about overcoming my problem?" Write what you said. Write how He responds.

At the end of the dialogue, ask God to give you a plan to move your mountain. With God, nothing is hopeless.

Join your prayer partner or another person if your partner is gone. Talk about how this might work in everyday life. What should you guard against? In what ways should you be proactive?

Romans 7: 17-20 MSG —"But I need something more! For if I know the law but still can't keep it, and if the power of sin within me keeps sabotaging my best intentions, obviously I need help! I realize I don't have what it takes, I can will it, but I can't do it. I decide to do good, but I don't really do it; I decide not to do bad, but then I do it anyway. My decisions, such as they are, don't result in actions. Something has gone wrong deep within me and gets the better of me every time."

Note: For more understanding of this, review "The God Connection" in the Principles section.

Pray the following prayers on your own or with your partner. Wait for what God tells you. Have your partner write down what God tells you in your notebook.

"Father God, What lie am I believing about my problem?"

"Father God, when is the first time I felt this way?"

If He shows you a time or situation, pray this prayer about whoever was in that circumstance.

"I choose to forgive _____ for _____."

Using the things you forgave that person for, pray the next prayer.

"God I renounce the lie that you will treat me the same way or make me feel the same way, such as _____."

"Now God, what is Your truth?"

His truth is always the most important part. Partners, be sure to write this part down. If you are doing this by yourself, be sure to record His truth.

"God, I surrender my weakness for _____ to You. I ask for Your power to be activated in my life so that I want do Your will instead of mine. Thank You for revealing to me how You have already begun to move the mountain in my life. Show me how worthwhile I am in Your eyes. Lead me to a path of life, instead of death."

Be sure to share your contact information with your partner and plan to text or call to support each other.

SHARE AND SING

Come together as a large group. Ask individuals to share anything they learned.

Song: Play "The Sound That Saved Us All" by Anthony Skinner (or another song of your choosing). Join hands, listen and commune with God asking Him to reveal to you anything else He has to say.

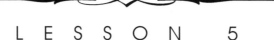

L E S S O N   5

CONTROL

THINK ABOUT IT

Do you have an issue with control which keeps you in a tailspin?

Do you have the opposite problem and give your control over to everyone else?

Who or what controls your life? Have you willingly allowed this control?

Who would you like to control your life?

READ AND WRITE

Philippians 2:9-11 NLT—"God elevated Him to the place of highest honor and gave Him the name above all other names, that at the name of Jesus every knee should bow, in heaven and on earth and under the earth, and every tongue declare that Jesus Christ is Lord, to the glory of God the Father."

Do you believe Jesus is the one who should have control of your life and deserves to be worshiped? How do you or should you show this in your daily life?

Ask God: In what areas do I take on a role that is not mine? In what ways do I refuse to take control when I know I should? How can I surrender any and all of these to You?

CREATE AND ACT

Take a sheet of paper and cut or rip it into strips of paper. On the strips of paper do the following,

Write down each role you are ready to surrender control of to the Lord.

Note: Every role we take on should be surrendered to Him. If there is one you are hesitant about surrendering, write it in your journal and come back to it later, asking God why you don't want to surrender it.

Write down each role you have refused to take control of, but know you should, and are now ready to surrender that to God's bidding.

Once you are done read each one aloud and ask the Lord to take on that role and take control of that area of your life. It can be something you are giving up control of to the Lord or something you need to take control of with the Lord's help.

After you ask the Lord to take that role and help you, fold the strip of paper in half and ask Him a new way to look at that role. Write what He says on the paper.

EXAMPLES

I am a child of the one true God.

I am a follower of Jesus Christ.

I am loved.

I am cherished.

I am strong.

I am an overcomer.

I am victorious.

I am more than a conqueror.

I am allowed to enjoy life.

I am beautiful.

I am a daughter of the king.

I am self-sufficient in Christ's sufficiency.

I am understanding.

I am joy-filled.

I am loving.

Post these new roles around the space where you live. As you go about your day, take time to say aloud your new roles.

If you don't know if you have an issue of control or lack of control, ask God. If you sense you do, ask God to show you the earliest time this occurred. (Review The God Connection in the Principles section.)

Whoever was involved in that situation, say out loud to God, "I forgive ____(the person)_____ for _____(how they made you feel such as making me feel I had to be in charge or that I couldn't control anything)_____."

If the situation involved a sibling or peer, you will speak to Jesus for the next part. If it involved your earthly dad or a father figure, you will speak to Father God. If it involved your mom or a mother figure, you will speak to the Holy Spirit.

Say out loud, "Jesus, I renounce the lie that you make me feel _____." (You are renouncing the same feeling your siblings or peers made you feel. Be specific, just like Teresa demonstrated in the book.)

Next, ask Jesus, "What is Your truth?" You just asked the God of the universe a question. He will answer. We just have to be aware of the answer. A picture might float across the big scene of your mind or a movie. You might sense something like a feeling of peace. You might hear a word or a sentence. Don't overthink this. Don't try to put thoughts in your mind. Whatever you sense, see or hear will likely be your answer.

Write down the truth He gives you. Then look up scriptures that correspond to the truth He gave you. The true test of whether this is from God or not will be if it aligns with Scripture.

Do some large group sharing. Just ask the participants, "Does anyone want to share what just happened to them?"

SING AND PRAY

Song: Play, "In Over My Head (Crash Over Me)" by Bethel Music and Jenn Johnson. Find the lyrics from the internet. Print them out for each participant. They can sing along or just ponder the words. Go from this directly to praying with partners. Ask them to share with their partners how they can view being in over their heads differently. How can that feeling lead you to a closer relationship with Jesus?

1 John 5:18-19 NIV—"We know that anyone born of God does not continue to sin; the One who was born of God keeps them safe, and the evil one cannot harm them. We know that we are children of God, and the whole world is under the control of the evil one."

Pray with your partner about what God showed you during this session. Ask Him to take complete control of your life. Surrender again anything you have been trying to control or trying to not control, but should.

"Loving Jesus, thank you for keeping me safe from the evil one. For so long, I have tried to control my own destiny and it has been exhausting. No matter how hard I try, I cannot overcome the temptations of the world on my own. Please take control of my life. Lead me to overcome the addictions and sins I struggle with. I know You have great plans for my life. Right now, I surrender all that I am to all that You are. I give You control of every part of me. I am ready to do the difficult work of transformation—body, soul and spirit. Transform me. Make me new so I can step into the destiny You have for me. Thank You for Your sweet grace. Amen."

Leaders: Remind group members to share contact information with their partner and stay in touch during the week.

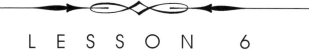

SHAME

THINK ABOUT IT

When do you have feelings of shame?

What do you do to avoid feeling shame?

Do you feel there is a wall of shame in your life?

READ AND WRITE

Ephesians 2:10 TPT— "We are God's poetry, a recreated people who will fulfill the destiny He has given each of us for we are joined to Jesus, the Anointed One. Even before we were born God planned in advance our destiny and the good works we would do to fulfill it."

What does it mean to you to be God's poetry?

How do you become recreated if you've already been made new once at salvation?

What destiny does Jesus have for you and how can you step into what He's already planned for you before you were even born?

Can you thwart His destiny? How?

Have you done this? In what way?

Proverbs 13:19 TPT—"When God fulfills your longing, sweetness fills your soul."

What do you long for? How do your longings impact your life?

How can God be true sweetness for your soul?

What would it look like for Him to fill your soul with sweetness?

CREATE AND ACT

Leaders: Hand out paper and pens if necessary or have them use a piece of notebook paper they can remove from their notebook. Ask them to get in a place where they feel comfortable writing honestly. Some may want more privacy than others. If doing personal study, find a quiet place to reflect your own.

Write down all the reasons you feel shame now. Write down all the reasons or times you felt shame in the past.

Ask God: "What is the first time I felt shame, the earliest moments in my life?" Write that down.

Ask members to join their partners and go through The God Connection Process regarding that situation. Each partner should help lead the other through the Process. Do this on your own if doing the personal study or with an accountability partner.

Whoever was involved in the earliest situation, have the partner say out loud to God, "I forgive ____(the person)_____ for _____(how they made you feel such as making me feel ashamed, ridiculed, abused, be specific)_____." (Continue through The God Connection Process in the Principles section.)

Allow the other partner to do the same.

Be sure to ask God, "What is Your truth?" Have your partner write that down on a blank page in your notebook.

Beside each shame write a truth you know God would give you. Such as: I am redeemed, I am beautiful, God loves me, He holds me, I am His Child.

After each finishes, gather as a large group. Put a large trash can in the middle.

Say, "Now you are ready rip up your reasons for feeling shame. Renounce these reasons for shame as the lies they are. Speak the truth about who you are out loud. You may go through your entire list or you may do it one at a time. Then go over to the trash can and rip up the lists."

Song: Play "Glorious Ruins" by Hillsong softly in the background when renouncing the reasons for shame and speaking the truth. You will need to lead the way in doing this.

"The feeling that I am not enough is a lie. I am a child of God."

"I renounce the lie that I have sinned too much to be redeemed, I know that Jesus died on the cross to take away my sins."

"It is a lie that I am too far gone. I know God's grace is all I need. It is enough. No one is ever too far away for God to reach."

Note: If there seems to be hesitancy in accepting what God has told you, there may be a wall between you and the person of God with whom you are speaking. You may need to ask a different Person of the Trinity to help you remove the wall. In Teresa's case she asked Father God to help remove the wall between her and Jesus.

Simply ask, "Father God is there a wall between Jesus and me?" If you sense there is, ask Him, "Father, will you show me the wall?" It could be anything. Teresa's was a donut wall. Ask God if He will tear it down or if you and He can tear it down. You may have to do some things to be ready to remove the wall. Some walls are meant for protection. Ask God if you are ready to remove the wall. When you are ready cooperate with Him for the removal. (Review the section "Barriers" in the Principles section.)

SHARE

Romans 8:1-2 NIV—"Therefore, there is now no condemnation for those who are in Christ Jesus because through Christ Jesus the law of the Spirit who gives life has set you free from the law of sin and death."

Leaders: Have the members sit in a circle and bow their heads. Ask them to picture handing their shame to Jesus. Have them picture Him accepting their shame and giving them His truth in exchange.

SING AND PRAY

Ask them to stand and worship believing what God believes about them.

Song: Play "Still Saving Me" by Dave Fitzgerald" or Bethel Music.

Close with a prayer reiterating how God feels about each person.

"Thank You Jesus for saving me. Thank You that You're still saving me. Thank You that despite all I've done, You still call me beautiful. You are a faithful God who never fails. Whatever You've started in me, You say it will be completed. Thank You for opening my eyes to Your kindness that leads me to Your truth. I love You, Lord. I'm so glad that You accept me, shame and all. You don't call me names like I call myself. You, oh God, You call me beautiful. Help me to do the same. In Jesus' name. Amen."

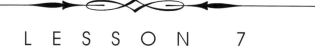

L E S S O N   7

UNACCEPTED

THINK ABOUT IT

Do you feel whole in your body? Why or why not?

Do you feel whole in your soul? Why or why not?

Do you feel whole in your Spirit? Why or why not?

How do you feel about God? Do you see him as a Father figure who wants the best for you? As someone who wants to control you with lots of rules? As someone who is angry when you fail to live up to his expectations?

READ AND WRITE

Isaiah 43:1 NIV—"Do not fear, for I have redeemed you; I have summoned you by name; you are Mine."

What would be different in your life if you really believed you have been redeemed by God and that He accepts you with all your imperfections? How would your daily life change? How would it change if you felt someone else did not accept you, but you knew God did?

Acts 10:34-35 MSG—"Peter fairly exploded with his good news: 'It's God's own truth, nothing could be plainer: God plays no favorites! It makes no difference who you are or where you're from—if you want God and are ready to do as he says, the door is open.'"

How do you know that you believe God accepts you as you are right now? Has there ever been a time you feel God plays favorites? Write about that and how you felt.

How does God see you? What words would He use to describe you? List these. Find Scriptures which verify how God sees you.

Psalm 139:14 NIV—"I praise you because I am fearfully and wonderfully made; your works are wonderful, I know that full well."

What does this verse say about how and why God accepts you?

In what ways are you relying on yourself, instead of God, to feel whole?

2 Corinthians 3:18 AMP—"And we all, with unveiled face, continually seeing as in a mirror the glory of the Lord, are progressively being transformed into His image from one degree of glory to even more glory, which comes from the Lord, who is the Spirit."

The wonderful thing about God's acceptance of us is He doesn't leave us there. He continues to work with us progressively transforming us—body, soul and spirit. What specifically does it look like in your life to allow the Lord to change you from glory to even more glory?

CREATE AND ACT

In your journal, make three columns. In the first column list brief statements to help you remember times in your life that you were wounded by what other people said or did that left you feeling unaccepted. Keep going until you have them all listed.

In the next column, write a statement that describes how you felt. Example: ugly, not good enough, small, insignificant, dumb, a blob, angry, frustrated, sad.

Ask Jesus, what is the truth about me? Write His truth in the third column.

If you are having trouble understanding His truth, ask Him, "What do You think of me, Jesus?" Essentially, this is what we want to understand. What is Jesus' truth about me?

Leaders: Ask the members to form two lines. On your start command, they will hug the woman across from them and share one of God's truths with them. Don't worry if it is a truth you remember that God shared with them. Just share a truth God gave you or one God is prompting you to share with them. Now change partners. Do the same. Continue the process until everyone has shared with every person.

If doing the study by yourself, find someone you know feels unaccepted and give him or her one of God's truths for you. For instance, go up to the person, hug them and whisper in their ear, "God loves you" or some other truth.

SHARE, SING AND PRAY

2 Corinthians 5:17 NLT—"This means that anyone who belongs to Christ has become a new person. The old life is gone; a new life has begun!"

God accepts us and changes us at the same time.

Do some group or partner sharing: Of the words God used to describe you, what are the ones which are most meaningful to you and why?

Song: Play "How He Loves Us" by Marc James or another song about God's love. Play this song standing in a circle holding hands. Ask the women to think about how Jesus loves and accepts them and has a wonderful plan for their lives.

Pray for each other being sure to include the ways God accepts each of you. A sample prayer is below.

"Dear Lord, thank You for creating my friend and accepting her for who she is. Please help her to forgive herself for all the ways she feels she falls short of who You call her to be. Thank You for creating her to be a _____ woman. Thank you for giving her new life. Please show her the wonderful life You have planned for her."

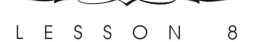

L E S S O N   8

HUNGER

SING

Song: Play "We Are Hungry" by Kathryn Scott. Find the lyrics and print copies for each participant. Ask them to sing along.

Afterwards ask the group: "How can we be as hungry for Jesus as we are for certain foods?" What would that look like?

If doing the study by yourself, ask yourself that question and journal about it.

THINK ABOUT IT

What did you inherit from your family?

What temptations did you inherit from your family?

Where did you learn your relationship with food?

How can the Holy Spirit as the Comforter comfort you as much as your favorite comfort food?

READ AND WRITE

John 6:35 NIV—"Then Jesus declared, 'I am the bread of life. Whoever comes to Me will never go hungry, and whoever believes in Me will never be thirsty.'"

Who or what sustains you?

How can Jesus fulfill your hunger and your thirst?

Is He telling the disciples to eat Him and drink Him? What is His meaning here?

John 14:27 AMP—"Peace I leave with you; My perfect peace I give to you; not as the world gives do I give to you. Do not let your heart be troubled, nor let it be afraid. Let My perfect peace calm you in every circumstance and give you courage and strength for every challenge."

Who or what gives you peace?

What barriers are holding you back from feeling peace?

CREATE AND ACT

List one of your favorite comfort food recipes. Why is it your favorite? What memories does it bring up when you cook it or eat it?

Find a way to make a healthier version of this recipe. You can look online if you need to. For instance, substitute almond flour or other flours for wheat flour. Substitute stevia, mashed bananas, honey or agave for sweetener. Actually make the recipe.

After you make the recipe, invite over your family and friends (if possible) to share your new creation. Prepare it for your next family get-together or party with friends. Print out the recipe and bring it to your group meeting. Or find a recipe on the internet and bring that.

WHERE DID YOU LEARN YOUR RELATIONSHIP WITH FOOD?

Go back to the Think About It section at the beginning of the chapter. If you haven't already, answer the question, "Where did I learn my relationship with food?" Understand this relationship was formed early in your life from your mother or father or caregivers standing in for your mother or father.

Your relationship with food may have been nothing like Teresa's. It may have been one that downplayed food or controlled food and made you want it even more. Just ask yourself the question and see what God shows you. In either case, it is not God's best for you.

When we realize we have an unhealthy relationship with food and it stems from someone we love, we may have trouble forgiving them. To forgive them sounds like they did something wrong. Actually, it's the way we perceived it. But, the child within us is still emotionally connected to that perception. As such, that emotion governs how we feel about food and many times is the reason we feel we can't give it up because it feels like we are dishonoring our relatives whom we love dearly.

On the flip side, our relationship with a matriarch may have been one where she was trying to control what we ate in order to teach us healthy eating principles. However, we rebelled against that and as adults found ourselves overindulging even though we didn't want to. We may have rationalized she didn't do anything wrong, and therefore we don't need to forgive her.

The child within us was affected emotionally. She either wanted to eat everything in sight to feel the comfort she felt from her mother figure, or she was rebelling and eating everything she wanted because she didn't like what her mother figure, the teacher, taught her.

In each of these situations, the mother figure did nothing wrong. The little child within us, though, caught on to an emotion. In order to release the emotion, we must go through the process of forgiveness.

Some of the roles of the mother are to comfort and teach us. These are also some of the Holy Spirit's roles. He is called Comforter and Teacher.

THE GOD CONNECTION

If it was a mother figure where you learned your relationship with food, go through The God Connection Process. (Review the Principles section for help.) Forgiving your mother figure, and renounce the lies Holy Spirit will treat you that way and won't comfort you with what lasts or won't teach you how to avoid temptations. Then, hear His truth.

Some individuals learn their relationship with food from a father figure or even a sibling. If this is true for you, go through The God Connection process forgiving the father figure and renouncing lies and hearing truth from Father God or doing the same with your sibling and Jesus.

SHARE

Share with your partner about whom you needed to forgive and why. If doing the study on your own, journal about this.

Philippians 4:11-13 TPT—"I have learned to be satisfied with whatever I have. I know what it means to lack and I know what it means to experience overwhelming abundance. For I'm trained in the secret of overcoming all things, whether in fullness or in hunger. And I find the strength of Christ's explosive power infuses me to conquer every difficulty."

How does going to a family dinner or a place where your favorite food is served make you feel? Journal about this and then share with your partner or the group. Pray together asking God to forgive those who helped you form unhealthy relationships with food.

Ask yourself, what legacy am I leaving for my family when I cook unhealthy foods? What can I do to leave a better legacy? What traditions do we currently have that do not center around food? What traditions could we create? Write these down.

Ask God to help you create new memories for yourself and your family not based around food. Ask Him to help you find satisfaction in your relationship with Him.

Share your thoughts about this with your partner or with the group. Understand this piece is vital on your healthy living, total transformation journey.

SING AND PRAY

Song: Play "Christ Is Enough" by Hillsong Live.

Leaders: Ask the members to think about in what ways He is enough for them.

After the song is over, ask the members to share the ways in which Christ is enough or you want to believe He is enough for you.

"Holy Spirit, You are the Great Comforter. Please help me to forgive my family for any relationship with food or temptations I may have inherited. Help me to create new memories based around You, rather than around temptations which will kill me if I continue to indulge in them. Fill the hunger in my soul with Your love. Please help me to be like Paul in his letter to the Philippians and find satisfaction in You, no matter the circumstance. I lay my weakness, my addiction, at Your feet. I need Your strength to face temptation. Give me Your power to become an overcomer. Amen."

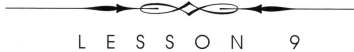

L E S S O N   9

MOVE

SING

Song: Play "Running" by Hillsong Live. Run or walk around the room as it plays. Begin a group discussion using the "Think About It" questions.

THINK ABOUT IT

How did you feel about exercise when you were a child?

Was there any exercise you enjoyed doing or any active play you enjoyed, such as swimming, biking, hiking, playing ball?

How does the thought of exercise make you feel?

Is there any exercise you enjoy doing today?

How do you feel after exercising?

Do you regularly exercise? If not, what's holding you back?

READ AND WRITE

1 Corinthians 9:24-27 NIV—"Do you not know that in a race all the runners run, but only one gets the prize? Run in such a way as to get the prize. Everyone who competes in the games goes into strict training. They do it to get a crown that will not last, but we do it to get a crown that will last forever. Therefore I do not run like someone running aimlessly; I do not fight like a boxer beating the air. No, I strike a blow to my body and make it my slave so that after I have preached to others, I myself will not be disqualified for the prize."

In what ways do you have control over your body?

Will you be disqualified for the prize of eternal life? If so, why?

Hebrews 12:1-2 MSG—"Strip down, start running—and never quit! No extra spiritual fat, no parasitic sins. Keep your eyes on Jesus, who both began and finished this race we're in. Study how He did it. Because he never lost sight of where He was headed—that exhilarating finish in and with God."

What do you need to strip out of your life so you can start running with Jesus towards God?

CREATE AND ACT

Create a start-stop plan for yourself. Write it out in your journal.

What is one thing you want to stop doing?

What is one thing you can do in its place?

How is your stop-start SMART? This means how is it specific, measurable, attainable, realistic and timely? Write out how each meets that criteria.

How are you going to keep yourself accountable for starting this new healthy habit?

Schedule your start-stop plan into your daily life.

Set a reminder or an appointment on your phone or in your calendar.

Find ways to remind you of what you are doing.

Don't think about your stop. Simply put boundaries around that thing. For instance, Teresa says she envisions electric fences around the things she has stopped. If your stop comes into your mind, take that thought captive by focusing on your start and how healthy it makes you feel.

Think about your start. Meditate on it. Remember it. Say things like, "I get to eat healthy. I choose to eat healthy. I love my exercise time. I look forward to feeling wonderful when I eat right and exercise."

Ask someone else to start this new habit with you. Share your start-stop with the people in your life.

PRAY AND SHARE

Deuteronomy 30:19-20 NLT—"Today I have given you the choice between life and death, between blessings and curses. Now I call on heaven and earth to witness the choice you make. Oh, that you would choose life, so that you and your descendants might live! You can make this choice by loving the Lord your God, obeying him, and committing yourself firmly to Him."

God so badly wants you to choose life. He has great plans for you if only you will let Him lead You. He is the only one who can break your addictions and give you life, but you have to let Him. You have to choose life.

CHOOSE A LIFE VERSE

To solidify your desire to choose life and go in God's direction, choose a Scripture which speaks to you and your life purpose. Ask God to recall to your mind a verse which speaks about who you are and what He made you to do. What do you want to do? What is the desire of your heart? You can google scriptures about life purpose or plans or God's will or any subject you are interested in such as teaching, healing, prophecy, music, leadership.

Find a verse and make it your life verse. Write it in your journal. Write a brief statement about why you are choosing this verse to direct your life.

Note: You can always change your life verse. This verse may direct you for a season until God gives you a new one to direct you.

Share your life verse and your stop-start with your partner. Share the ways you are choosing life. Then if you feel led to choose life, pray from your heart about how you are choosing life. A sample prayer is listed below, but in reality a prayer straight from your heart is the very best.

"Father God, I know I am a sinner who struggles with temptation. I can't overcome these addictions on my own. Thank you for your grace and mercy. Today, I choose life! I don't want my temptations to lead me down the path towards death anymore. I choose blessings instead of curses. Please help me to obey your loving will. I commit myself fully to you today. I want to run my race for you and your kingdom. I love you God!"

SHARE

On a blank piece of paper write your life verse, adding any special touches to it.

Leaders: Bring paper and colored markers to use for this. Then invite each one to bring their life verses with them and form a circle. Go around the circle and ask each to share their verse with the entire group. If they wish, they may also share their stop-start.

SING

Song: Play "Amazed" by the Desperation Band. Ask the members to join in singing. This is a simple easy-to-learn song. Play it on repeat if you wish. Just worship. This is a time of commitment to seal the decisions they have made in this session.

L E S S O N   1 0

UNPROTECTED

THINK ABOUT IT

What areas of your life do you feel safe and protected?

What areas of your life do you feel vulnerable and unprotected?

Who or what provides you with protection?

READ AND WRITE

1 John 4:4 NKJV—"You are of God, little children, and have overcome them, because He who is in you is greater than he who is in the world."

In what ways does God protect you? How big is the devil compared to God?

John 14:27 NIV—"Peace I leave with you; My peace I give you. I do not give to you as the world gives. Do not let your hearts be troubled and do not be afraid."

When you are afraid what calms you? Be honest.

CREATE AND ACT

Make a list of all the situations that made you feel vulnerable and unprotected as a child. (If you're having trouble remembering, try using your non-dominant hand to write.) Next to each situation, write what made you feel protected or comforted as a child.

As an adult what causes you to feel vulnerable and unprotected? How would you provide comfort for yourself in the midst of that situation?

Are there any similarities between your two lists from when you were a child to when you were an adult?

What do you turn to for security and protection now? Does it actually help you feel more secure? Is it a lasting sense of security? Is it healthy for your life and the lives of those around you?

Jesus wants us to turn to Him in all things, big or small, in times of contentment or fear. He even sent us the ultimate Comforter, the Holy Spirit.

EXCHANGE

Hand to Jesus each thing you have turned to for courage, comfort, well-being or protection. Ask Him to forgive you for not turning to Him first. For each thing you hand Him, ask Jesus, "What do you give me in exchange?" In your journal, write down each thing you handed Him and what He gave you in exchange. (Review Exchanges in the Principles section.)

As an adult, where do you feel uncovered, unprotected or vulnerable? Do you feel Father God can and will protect you from any and everything? Will He protect you from yourself? Whatever is the biggest area of concern, ask Father God, "When is the first time I felt this concern?" Journal about the incident. Who was involved? How did it make you feel?

Regarding that specific incident, ask Jesus, "Where were You during that difficult time in my life? (Use one specific time, such as how I did in this chapter when I felt a panic attack or as a child when I didn't know where He was during difficult times growing up.) Write down what He says.

Share with your partner how that makes a difference to you or journal about it if doing the study alone.

Do you believe God is able to provide protection, comfort and security for you?

PRAY AND SHARE

2 Timothy 1:7 NKJV—"For God has not given us a spirit of fear, but of power and of love and of a sound mind."

What does it mean that God has given us a spirit of power, love and a sound mind? How can these things overcome our fears?

Close the meeting by thanking God for giving us a spirit of power, love and a sound mind. Pair off with someone. Stand facing each other. Each of you one at a time should touch the other person on the shoulder and say, "I bless you with God's spirit of power, love and a sound mind." Now, find another and do the same thing. Continue until you have blessed everyone. Pray other blessings over individuals as you are led.

SING AND PRAY

Song: Play "No Longer A Slave" by Jonathan David and Melissa Helser or Bethel Music. Worship together.

"Thank You, Lord, for overcoming the darkness that has invaded the world. Thank You for bringing light and overcoming all my fears. Please help me turn to You when I am afraid. Reveal to me how You want to use the spirit of power, love and a sound mind for Your glory! Help me turn to You in times of trouble and temptation. Help me not to be afraid, but to rely on You to give me peace and courage to overcome the darkness that surrounds me. Help me remember every minute that You split the seas so I can walk right through them. I know You rescued me. I am standing right now and saying, 'I am a child of God. I'm no longer a slave to fear.'"

Ask the group to say that with you. "I am a child of God. I'm no longer a slave to fear."

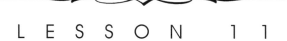

L E S S O N 1 1

GREED

THINK ABOUT IT

In what ways are you greedy?

Who do you rely on to provide for you?

Do you trust Father God will provide for you?

READ AND WRITE

1 Thessalonians 5:24 NIV—"The One who calls you is faithful, and He will do it."

How has God provided in your life so far?

Ephesians 2:10 TPT—"We have become His poetry, a recreated people that will fulfill the destiny He has given each of us, for we are joined to Jesus, the Anointed One. Even before we were born, God planned in advance our destiny and the food works we would do to fulfill it."

In what ways have you become His poetry, masterpiece or handiwork as other versions translate this verse?

In what way have you been recreated?

How have you seen God working in your life?

Do you believe Father God has a destiny for you?

CREATE AND ACT

In your journal, draw a picture using colored pencils, markers or crayons of who Father God is to you. Put yourself in the picture. What size are you in relation to God and He to you? Where is Father God in relationship to you? How far or close? What is His posture? What is yours? Can you see His face? What is the look on His face? Do you see colors? What colors? What feeling do you have in His presence? Put as much of this as you can in your picture.

Ask Father God, "Is there a lie I am believing about You?" He may tell you the lie or you may have a sense of the lie just looking at the picture. Write the lie on the picture somewhere.

Ask Father God, "What is the truth?" When He gives you the truth, if it changes your picture, draw a second picture depicting the truth and write it on that picture. He may give you a truth about the first picture you drew so that you see it in a different way. If so, cross out the lie and write the truth on that picture.

In this time of truth giving ask Father God, "In what way do I need to trust You to be my provider?" Write down what He says. If you don't understand His answer, ask Him to teach you how to trust Him more.

As a group, hold out your hands and symbolically place in your hands the thing you think you don't have enough of whether it is time, food, strength, love, relationships, wisdom, courage or anything else.

Now together as a group, say, "Father God I give you my not enough. What do you give me in exchange?" As your leader tells you to do so, speak out loud what He gave you. Be sure to write it in your journal.

PRAY

Ephesians 1:7-8 GW—"Through the blood of his Son, we are set free from our sins. God forgives our failures because of his overflowing kindness. He poured out his kindness by giving us every kind of wisdom and insight."

It doesn't matter if we fail because God forgives our failures. I hand Him my selfishness and He gives me more than enough. God always trades up.

In small or large groups depending on what time you have, share what God gave you when you gave Him your not enough and how that made you feel.

Then, pray in popcorn fashion about what you are thankful for. Just pray out loud saying what you are thankful for. You can pray as many times as you like, but just say one thing at a time.

If there are five in your group you may have 30 things or more you are thankful for. Just continue until you are done. If doing the study on your own, list these and then pray, thanking God for each thing.

SING AND CLOSE

Song: Play "Jesus Loves Me" and/or "Good, Good Father" by Chris Tomlin. Have the lyrics available for the group to sing together. Encourage them to feel the words and react to them by moving, raising their hands, kneeling or whatever they wish.

"Thank You, Jesus, for laying down Your life for me, even though I did nothing and can do nothing to deserve Your sacrifice. Thank You, God, for Your grace, even though I have failed You and will never deserve Your love. Please help me in all circumstances to feel I have enough because You are enough. I don't need worldly things to fill up my life. I just need You. Thank You for being enough! Amen."

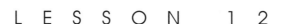

L E S S O N   1 2

DECEPTION

THINK ABOUT IT

How have you experienced hell in your own life?

Did you feel powerless to stop your personal hell?

How have you experienced heaven in your life?

Is the heaven you experienced something God created, or something the world convinced you was heaven, but actually hurt you? If it was something that misled you, how were you deceived?

In what ways do you feel God's presence in your life?

READ AND WRITE

John 8:42 NIV—"Jesus said to them, 'If God were your Father, you would love me, for I have come here from God. I have not come on my own; God sent me. Why is my language not clear to you? Because you are unable to hear what I say.'"

Do you love Jesus with all your heart, or do you find it hard to surrender? If you are having trouble surrendering completely, look at the next verse:

John 8:44 NIV—"You belong to your father, the devil, and you want to carry out your father's desires. He was a murderer from the beginning, not holding to the truth, for this is no truth in him. When he lies, he speaks his native language, for he is a father and the father of lies."

What lies have you believed from the father of lies?

John 8:51 NIV—"Very truly I tell you, whoever obeys my word will never see death."

Whom would you rather obey: the father of lies, or the One who sacrificed Himself so we could live with Him for all eternity?

Name some times the devil has deceived you. How long did it take you to recognize the deception?

How does the devil operate in your life? Does he overtly deceive you or is he more covertly deceptive?

List the times he deceived you. How did God reveal truth in each situation?

How is he deceiving you in regard to food issues in your life?

CREATE AND ACT

Ask God, "What lies am I believing about the foods I eat or have eaten?" In your journal title your page, "Beliefs and

Truths About Food". Create three columns. Label them Food, Beliefs and Truths.

Under Food write your favorite foods, unhealthy foods and what you consider healthy foods.

In the Beliefs column, write the things you believe about that food. For instance, beside my great-grandma's oatmeal cake, I'd write, "I can't live without this." Beside salad, I might have written (in days past), "I can't stand salad."

In your column of beliefs, stop at each one and ask God, "Where did I learn this? Is it a lie or a truth?" Write down His answer in the second column next to your belief.

WHAT IS YOUR TRUTH, GOD?

Go down the column again and ask God, "What is Your truth about this food?" Write His answers in the last column.

Take some time to think about the lies God showed you, the source of those lies and the truths. Do you see any trends among your lists?

Go through The God Connection Process with any of the situations which seem overwhelming or unbelievable to you. You may want to do this with each situation making sure you understand and accept the truth God gave you.

Ask God to show you what heaven is actually like. Illustrate this by writing a poem, short story or description.

As part of your daily prayer time, reflect on the image of heaven God revealed to you. Ask God to help you find His heaven on earth, not the one the world or you have created. Ask Him to guide your life so that as Jesus promised you will never have to see death, which means spending eternity in hell.

PRAY

Revelation 21:25-27 —"On no day will its gates ever be shut, for there will be no night there. The glory and honor of the nations will be brought into it. Nothing impure will ever enter it, nor will anyone who does what is shameful or deceitful, but only those whose names are written in the Lamb's book of life."

The evil one does not like for us to think about spending eternity in heaven. Spend some time meditating on heaven. Ask God to show you what heaven is really like. Think about what it means when Jesus said in Matthew 6:10, "Your kingdom come. Your will be done on earth as it is in heaven."

Placing your chairs in a circle, in popcorn fashion have the members say in one word what they feel heaven will be like.

SING AND CLOSE

Stand, hold hands and play a favorite song about heaven, depending on your taste in music. You could play "I Can Only Imagine" by Mercy Me or an old song about heaven, such as "I've Got A Mansion."

Close in prayer. "Lord, I know whatever I do will never be enough to inherit the majesty of heaven and eternity with You. You give us grace so that we never have to be apart from Your love. Thank you for sending your Son as a living sacrifice for my life, so that when I accept Him I can live with You forever!

"Please help me avoid the lies of the devil. I know You have already overcome him. I need Your help to recognize the times and places when he deceives me. Teach me how to listen to Your voice and Yours alone.

"Teach me how to quickly dismiss the lies the evil one whispers to me. Remind me to stand up to him and say, 'No, I will not do what you want me to do. I am a child of obedience to the Lord My God. You have no hold on me!'

"My one desire, Oh God, is to be your obedient child. Teach me how. Remind when I'm walking off the path. Show me the way You want me to walk. Amen."

UNANSWERED PRAYER

SING

Song: Play "How Great is Our God" by Chris Tomlin. Print lyrics and sing together.

THINK ABOUT IT

As a group discuss these questions: What is the miracle you have been praying for? Has this prayer been answered or does it seem like no one is listening?

Do you trust God will take care of you?

Do you try to fit the Bible into your life? Or do you try to fit your life into the Bible?

Do you do what the Bible tells you or do you pick and choose the parts you like?

Do you believe your struggles are bigger than God?

If you do what the Bible tells you, how does that affect your life? If you only choose the parts you like, are you willing to try looking at the whole Bible to guide your life?"

READ AND WRITE

Psalm 34:4 NKJV—"I sought the Lord, and He heard me, and delivered me from all my fears."

What do you want the Lord to deliver you from?

How have you sought the Lord's help?

Psalm 37:4 NKJV—"Delight yourself also in the Lord and He shall give you the desires of your heart."

What are the desires of your heart?

How can you delight yourself in the Lord?

CREATE AND ACT

Matthew 6:9-10 NIV—"Our Father in heaven, hallowed be Your name. Your kingdom come, Your will be done, on earth as it is in heaven."

How might God's will be different from your will for a certain situation?

In your journal, make a chart with three columns. Label these Problems, My Will, God's Will. Under problems, list difficulties you have taken to God or are currently praying about.

In the center column, write how you wanted them answered or how you currently are wanting them answered. This might include how you feel you'll know that the answer will come and the timing of it.

Under God's will write how God overcame these difficulties or answered this prayer. Notice how the way He answered prayers in the past is similar or different from the way you wanted it answered. Thank Him for answering the prayer according to His will and not yours. What might have happened if the prayer was answered in your will or way? How was His way better? If you can't see that, ask Him to reveal that to you.

Set aside time everyday to go down the list of prayer requests that still need to be answered. Humble your heart and ask Him to answer the prayer in His will and in His time. Tell Him You trust Him to take care of the problem. Ask Him to help you see things from heaven's perspective.

Keep track of how God works in your life by continuing to add to your list, and recording how God answers the prayers that are currently unanswered.

Post answered prayers some place where you can see them and remember God's faithfulness.

PRAY

1 John 5:14-15 NIV—"This is the confidence we have in approaching God: that if we ask anything according to His will, He hears us. And if we know that He hears us—whatever we ask—we know that we have what we asked of Him."

Play soft instrumental music through the prayer time. Share with your partner what you feel like is the most pressing need on your list of unanswered prayers. If you feel God will never answer it, share that honestly. Then, pray for each other's prayer requests and for God to give you the faith to believe He is in the process of answering your prayer.

Ask Him to help you see from heaven's perspective to get a better understanding of the bigger picture. Ask Him, "Am I really praying Your will be done or my will be done? Help me to be satisfied if Your will is different from mine. Change my will to line up with Your will." Be sure to write down what He says.

Spend some time praying in groups of four or five. Pray for one specific prayer for each person being sure to pray that His will be done.

SING AND SHARE

Stand in a circle. Play "Awesome In This Place" by Natalie Grant. Sing along.

Put a chair in the middle. Ask anyone who wishes to come forward, sit in the chair and share their prayer request. Have the women gather around her touching her and have one person pray out loud.

Close in a final group prayer.

"Thank You God that You do hear my prayers and You do answer them in Your way and time. I know there is no problem too big for You to handle in Your way and in Your time! Help me to follow You in all that I do and submit to Your will no matter what that looks like. Thank You for all the prayers You have already answered, even the ones I don't recognize as answers, and all the prayers You will answer."

ANGER

THINK ABOUT IT

Do you express your anger or hide it?

If you express anger, how do you express it? Do you yell? Do you calmly talk about it after you've cooled down?

If you hide it, do you hold on to it? In what ways does that affect you?

How did Jesus express anger? (John 2:13-17, Mark 11:15-18)

Is anger always bad?

What role might anger play in your life?

READ AND WRITE

John 14:26 KJV—"But the Comforter, which is the Holy Ghost, whom the Father will send in My name, He shall teach you all things, and bring all things to your remembrance, whatsoever I have said unto you."

What brings you comfort? Do you automatically go to the Holy Spirit or some other source, such as comfort foods to help you through negative emotions?

2 Corinthians 3:17 NLT—"For the Lord is the Spirit, and wherever the Spirit of the Lord is, there is freedom."

What is your relationship with the Holy Spirit like? Is He your comforter? Does He give you freedom? Or is He a mystical idea, which sounds nice, but you don't have a personal relationship with?

Put a picture of who the Holy Spirit is to you in your mind. Note: many people find it difficult to do this because we don't normally picture the Holy Spirit. You may get a feeling or sense of who He is. You may hear music? Just notice where He is and what He is. Where are you in relationship to Him? Can you see His face? What expression do you see? Where are you in relationship to Him? What feeling do you get from the picture?

Now ask the Holy Spirit, "Is there a lie I am believing about You?" If He gives you a lie, write it down. Then, ask, "What is Your truth?" write this down. Does it resonate with you? Do you understand what He is telling you? If not, ask Him to teach you. Write down anything He shows or tells you.

CREATE AND ACT

Write a letter to someone in your life you felt angry with when you were a child, perhaps a mother or father figure. This might be someone you couldn't tell or express the anger to at the time.

The anger might have been because of an incident or a string of incidents. You may feel you don't have a right to be angry because they were sick, died early, were absent because of work or hospitalization, because they were your elders and you weren't supposed to be angry with them or any number of things.

Now is the time for you to understand that anger and what it has done to you.

WRITE TWO LETTERS

Write the first letter in your dominant hand as your adult self with all your rational feelings.

Write another one in your non-dominant hand about how you felt as a child. It might begin, I'm angry because...

Ask God, "What has stuffing this anger done to me?" Write what He shows you or tells you.

The only way to stop creating the negative results of pent up anger is to admit the child within you is still angry and governing a portion of your emotions.

It is imperative that you forgive this person. It's not necessary to confront them in person. They may already be deceased, but that anger is still in charge of your emotions. In the Principles section, revisit Forgive Others. Then go through The God Connection Process choosing to forgive the person, renouncing the lie the corresponding member of the Godhead will treat you that way and hearing His truth.

Now, go to the door of fear in your mind. Check to see if it's open or closed. If it is open, ask God what is still holding the door open. Then, go back through The God Connection

Process to forgive the individual in that situation. (Review "Doors" in the Principles section.)

In your journal, write about how you feel now. Do you have a different perspective on fear? If you forgave someone, do you have a different perspective about him or her? How did you see them before? How do you see them now?

PRAY AND SHARE

Isaiah 9:4 TLB—"For God will break the chains that bind His people."

Song: "Break Every Chain" by Will Reagan and United Pursuit Band should be ready to be played.

Prophetic Prayer Activity—Stand in circle. Ask the women to raise their hands if they felt they were set free of anger or any other negative emotion. Ask if they want to seal the breaking of that emotion.

Have individuals or small groups stand in the middle and hold their hands out in front of them. Using a long rope, wrap it around their hands. Tell them, "I am going to play a song and when you feel the power of God, move your hands in an outward motion so the rope falls off, like you are breaking a chain. Others should stand behind them in support.

After the song plays through, ask any who felt they weren't set free, but wanted to be set free to come forward and do the same thing. Ask others to come behind them and pray quietly. If any are having difficulty, ask if you can lay your hands on them and pray. Continue to repeat the song until all have had a chance to do this activity.

Stand in circle. Leaders tell the group, "Let's celebrate our freedom tonight. Let's sing, raise our hands, move and worship the Lord in the way that lets Him know you are happy He allows you to walk in freedom tonight."

SING AND CLOSE

Song: Play or sing a song about freedom such as "He Set Me Free" by Connie Smith. Have a pianist play it or search YouTube for the Gaither rendition. Or use a contemporary song, such as "I Am Set Free" by All Sons and Daughters.

Leaders: Ask the members to pray the following prayer or a similar one after you.

"Dear Lord, thank You for breaking the chains that bind me. Lead me to understand how You want me to overcome my addictions nd temptations with Your help. Help me understant You are the only One who has the power to help me when I surrender to You. Holy Spirit, I know you are the only true Comforter. Right now I hand my anger to You. I can no longer hang on to it. It will overwhelm me. Holy Spirit, will You replace my anger with Your peace and Your comfort? If that is possible I want it more than anything.

"I praise you for caring enough about me and my problems that You choose to make my body Your dwelling place. I think You right now for Your comfort and Your peace. Remind me, Holy Spirit, whenever the anger tries to rise up again that I can come to You. Amen."

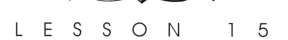

L E S S O N   1 5

PRETTY

SING

Song: Play "You Are So Beautiful" by Joe Cocker. Ask the group to sing along.

THINK ABOUT IT

Have you felt pretty in your life? Do you feel pretty now?

Have you felt smart in your life? Do you feel smart now?

What is God's truth about your beauty and intelligence?

READ AND WRITE

Song of Solomon 1:15 AMP—"Behold, you are beautiful, my love! Behold, you are beautiful. You have dove's eyes."

Do you believe that you are beautiful? Why or why not?

Do you believe God sees you as beautiful? Why or why not?

Isaiah 62:3 NLT—"The Lord will hold you in His hand for all to see—a splendid crown in the hand of God."

In what way does God treasure you so much that He sees you as a splendid crown?

What lies do you still need to overcome to see yourself with the same worth God sees?

CREATE AND ACT

Create two illustrations of yourself using words or pictures from magazines taped or glued onto construction paper. In the first one draw or describe yourself as you feel the world sees you or you see yourself. You can cut out photos and words from magazines along with written words to give the feel of how the world sees you or you see yourself. Be sure to put your name somewhere in the illustration.

In the second illustration, show how God sees you. What words does He use to describe you? What does He call you? How does God bring out the best in you? If you don't know, ask Him. How is God changing you from the inside out? Has God given you a new name? Be sure to put that in the illustration as well.

Now that you know how God sees you, how can you show this side of yourself to the world? Write specifics as to how you walk this out in your ordinary, every day life.

Leaders: In a large group, have each group member share their two illustrations and one thing they can do to show more of how God sees them.

SHARE

Colossians 3:12 NIV—"Therefore, as God's chosen people, holy and dearly loved, clothe yourself with compassion, kindness, humility, gentleness and patience. "

Leaders: It would be good to dim the lights for this exercise and have quiet instrumental music playing.

Form a Blessing Line. Divide your group in half. Have each group form a line facing the other with just enough space for someone to walk down the middle. The leader should stand at the beginning of the line facing the group. The line will move as one at a time each woman comes from the back of the line to where the leader is standing. The woman closes her eyes as the leader whispers a quick but meaningful word of encouragement, how she sees the individual, or a scripture.

The leader then turns her around. The woman puts her hands straight out to her sides (like an airplane or a T) and the first two women take her arms. First one whispers a word to her, then the next. They pass her to the next two women and so forth. Each set of women move her quickly to the end of the line whispering their words to her as she goes to the end of the line. She then takes her place to share with those coming down the line.

Before she gets to the end of the line, those at the end of the line should already be moving forward to go through. (You may want to have a helper tapping them on the shoulder to move forward for their time.)

This should move quickly with each woman giving one or two words to the one coming through the Blessing Line. The next woman should already be going through the line before the first one is finished. Continue until all the women have gone through the line. If you didn't get to share with someone, simply go up behind them in the line and whisper your words to her.

If you get lost in the travel, just make sure everyone has a chance through the line and has shared with others.

There are many variations of this such as placing a chair in the center of the room and having the rest of the women come by and whisper encouragement. When finished, the woman quickly gets up and the next woman sits down. Continue until all have had a chance. This works fine with a small group. The Blessing Line works better with a large group.

Leaders: This can be very emotional time for everyone. Have tissues available. Encourage the women to write what they remember from what was shared with them.

If you have time, do some sharing in the large group by answering the simple question, "How did you feel about what was shared with you?"

Personal Study: Ask God, "How do You see me?" Write down what He says and speak those blessings over yourself.

SING AND CLOSE

Song: Play "Still Saving Me" by Dave Fitzgerald.

Close in a group prayer/blessing. "Dear God, I bless the women here today with the ability to see themselves as you see them. Help them and me to act like Your daughters, princesses who You created us to reign with You. Help us even now to begin to understand what that looks like in our lives. Amen"

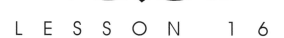

L E S S O N   1 6

PRIDE

THINK ABOUT IT

How do you feel about being feminine?

Are you afraid of your sexuality?

What do you fear about the person deep inside buried under excess weight?

Are you afraid of attracting the wrong kinds of men?

Are you afraid of being too prideful if you look too attractive?

Are you concerned you might be tempted to cheat on your husband or be promiscuous if you were too attractive?

Do you have any areas of your life where your actions are being led by your pride or your fear of seeming prideful?

What are you hiding from?

In what ways are you tempted?

How do you avoid temptation?

READ AND WRITE

John 16:33 NLT—"Here on earth you will have many trials and sorrows. But take heart, because I have overcome the world".

Jesus tells us He overcame the world. In what way do you need Him to help you overcome the world? Name one specific way a trial or temptation that plagues you?

Hebrews 4:15 NIV—"For we do not have a high priest who is unable to empathize with our weaknesses, but we have one who has been tempted in every way, just as we are—yet did not sin".

How did Jesus resist the temptations of this world?

Why do we fall short?

Romans 8:11 NIV—"And if the Spirit of Him who raised Jesus from the dead is living in you, He who raised Christ from the dead will also give life to your mortal bodies because of His Spirit who lives in you."

If we really understood this, how might this be a game-changer for us? When does He become powerful within me?

John 10:10 AMP—"The thief comes only in order to steal and kill and destroy. I came that they may have and enjoy life, and have it in abundance to the full, till it overflows."

What is abundance to you? What will it look like in your life?

Leaders: Fair warning, this next activity needs a lot of advance planning. And be sure to have your camera or camera phone ready. Some of my most cherished photos have come out of one of these great fun times.

CREATE AND ACT

This next activity really does go to some of the definition of abundance. It's party time! I'd like you to party WITHOUT food. If you do have food, make it be one your healthy alternatives, but watch portions.

For the rest of the session have a Girlie celebration party. Celebrate being a woman. There are several ways to do this. One of the most fun ways takes some advance planning. Announce several weeks ahead that you want women to bring fun dress up clothes, colorful robes, large dresses or lounging dresses, oversize jackets, shawls, boas, hats, wigs, sunglasses, large oversize sun glasses, costume jewelry, bangles, masks, even colorful table cloths can make great dress up clothes.

Put on some upbeat Christian music. Here's my playlist. Choose some of these or your own. You can go to YouTube and find each of these. "Wishful Thinking", "Move", "Shake" by Mercy Me; "Shackles" by Mary Mary; "Hold Me", "Beautiful Day" by Jamie Grace; "Miracle" by Moriah Peters; "Overcomer", "Stronger", "Joy Unspeakable" by Mandisa; "Alive", "Wake" by Hillsong Young & Free; "Gold" by Britt Nicole; "This Is The Stuff," "Free To Be Me", "Write Your Story", "He Knows My Name" by Francesca Batticelli; "Running" by Hillsong Live; "Me Without You," "Get Back Up", "Speak Life", "Feel It" by Toby Mac; "Awake My Soul (featuring LeCrae)", "God's Great Dance Floor" by Chris Tomlin. Or any Christian songs of any genre you wish to party with your girls and Jesus!

A more sedate thing to do would be to have a nail polish party. Ask women to bring a variety of polishes, even clear polish, nail files, clippers and manicure implements and enjoy doing each other's nails.

Be creative, if you have creative people. Play some upbeat Christian music and enjoy being girls! (Be careful with this. Nail polish can get messy. Use disposable tablecloths. You may want drop cloths under where you are sitting. Clean up the area no matter where you are.)

Personal Study: Plan a similar party inviting several close friends. Give them the rule of no unhealthy food. Be sure to define unhealthy as you perceive it.

SING AND CLOSE

Stand in a circle, join hands and sing along to "Beautiful Things" by Gungor.

Closing: Ask the members to find at least three others, look them in the eye and say, "You are beautiful."

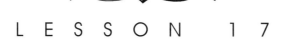

L E S S O N   1 7

FEAR

SING

Song: Play "Didn't I Walk On The Water" by Fresh Anointing. Be sure to print out the words to read or sing along. If working in a group, discuss the think about it questions.

THINK ABOUT IT

Do you trust Jesus?

In what areas do you need help trusting Jesus more?

Reflecting on areas that cause you to feel fear? When is the first time you felt this fear?

Is there someone you need to forgive who was involved in this root cause of fear? (Review The God Connection Process forgiving the person, renouncing the lie that a member of the Godhead will treat you that way and hear His truth.)

READ AND WRITE

1 John 4:18 NIV—"There is no fear in love. But perfect love drives out fear, because fear has to do with punishment. The one who fears is not made in perfect love."

How can the perfect love of Jesus drive out fear? If you still feel afraid, ask Jesus to show you His perfect love!

Psalm 91:5 NLT—"You will not fear the terror of night, nor the arrow that flies by day."

Why will we not fear these things?

CREATE AND ACT

We've dealt with many feelings going through this study. Of them all, real fear may be the biggest one. Many times we try to gloss over our fears. However, they affect us and limit our lives in profound ways. We have probably learned the verses that tell us not to fear. However, actually discarding fear takes digging deeper.

For this exercise, spread out around the room. Make sure you have a clean piece of paper. You can write front and back if you wish. Take some time to pray and ask the Lord, "What am I afraid of?" Begin writing a list of everything you are afraid of.

This list is just for you. It won't stay in your notebook. You won't have to reveal it to anyone unless you want to. We won't ask you to. We are going to do something profound with this list.

So write your list. Everything you've worried might happen is a fear. Every time someone abused you, yelled at you, hurt you in any way might be a fear. You might be afraid of snakes, mice, spiders or dogs. You might be afraid of flying, heights, being late, being early, being in crowds or being alone. You might be afraid of not having enough money to pay your bills, going bankrupt.

You might be afraid of dying, afraid others will die and leave you alone. You might be afraid of getting sick, of having a terminal illness or someone you love having the same. There are so many things we are afraid of.

I want you to spend some time on this. Let the hurts, pains, angers come out on your paper. Scream, cry, pound your fists, pace if you need to. Tonight, we are letting go of fear once and for all. But first we need to get it out where we can see what we are getting rid of. Don't let any hidden fear go unnoticed. We don't want any hangers on.

Tonight, fear has to go, in Jesus' name.

BURNING FEARS

Leaders: Play some quiet instrumental worship music. Five minutes may be enough time for them to write their fears, but don't rush it. Prepare a place to burn the paper the fears are written on. If you have access to area where you can build a bonfire, that is perfect. Perhaps there is a fireplace you can use.

Try bringing a hibachi and setting it on a patio away from the building. When all are ready ask the members to take their paper or papers with their fears written on them with them to where the fire is. Have the women come to the areas where the fears will be burned and form a half circle facing you.

Talk about the following.

We find many promises in God's Word regarding fear. Here are just a few of them.

Psalm 27:1 NKJV— "The LORD is my light and my salvation; Whom shall I fear? The LORD is the strength of my life; Of whom shall I be afraid?"

Psalm 34:4 NKJV— "I sought the LORD, and He heard me, And delivered me from all my fears."

This fire is symbolic of God delivering you from your fears. Tonight, He wants you to trust Him in the most intimate of ways. He wants you to trust Him with these things you've held on to. Your fears are protecting you from something you think will damage you.

Close your eyes right now and simply talk to Him and say, "Father God, I have mistakenly thought being afraid would protect me from these things. Tonight, I recognize only You can protect me. I need not be afraid of any of these things. You, Father God, are the strength of my life.

"I put all my hope and trust in You and You alone. I see now that fear has been a false protection in My life, even as food has been an equal culprit as a false comfort. I am ready now to give these fears completely to You. I have no use for them. I surrender them to You. As the smoke rises to Heavenward let it be a sweet aroma of my surrender to You."

When and if you are ready, feel free to come and burn your fears.

Song: Play "Oceans" by Hillsong as the members burn their fears. (Play it on repeat if additional time is needed for each person to have time to release these things which they have held on to for years. Burn your own list first and then be present to give them a hug after they burn their fears. Whisper words of encouragement.)

Personal Study: Invite some friends over and do this activity together or do it on your own. It can be powerful for you to mark this occasion alone or even with one other friend. Don't wait for someone to join you though. Releasing fears is something we all can do and should do before they overtake us.

SING AND PRAY

Psalm 91:4 NLT—"He will cover you with his feathers. He will shelter you with his wings. His faithful promises are your armor and protection."

Close your eyes and picture yourself safe within God's protection. Pray a prayer of thanksgiving for His promises and for His strength and watchcare over you.

Song: Play "Just Be Held," by Casting Crowns or "Sheltered Safe Within the Arms of God." The latter is an old hymn you can find on YouTube. If you have time play both.

"Dear Father God, thank You for Your protection. Please forgive me for not always trusting You and letting fear control me. Show me your perfect love so I can trust in you in all I do. Thank You for Your faithful promises that are my armor and protection. I know with Your Almighty strength I can be courageous and overcome every fear. Amen."

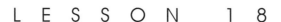

L E S S O N   1 8

INTIMACY

ASK

What is the number one problem, difficulty, personal problem, relationship or overwhelming burden you'd like to leave in this room tonight? I don't want you to tell anyone. I want you to just remember it. If doing a personal study, note this for yourself.

THINK ABOUT IT

Do you feel worthy of love? Why or why not?

Do you feel like you are enough, that you are accepted and loved just as you are?

Are you in an intimate relationship with another person? With Jesus?

READ AND WRITE

1 Samuel 16:7 NIV—"The Lord does not look at the things people look at. People look at the outward appearance but the Lord looks at the heart."

When the Lord looks at your heart, what does He see?

Mark 12:30-31 NLT—"And you must love the Lord your God with all your heart, all your soul, all your mind, and all your strength. The second is equally important: Love your neighbor as yourself. No other commandment is greater than these."

Which of these commandments is harder—loving God, loving your neighbor or loving yourself and why?

What do you need to change to follow these commandments?

John 15:4 TPT—"Step into life-union with Me for I have stepped into life-union with you. For as a branch severed from the vine will not bear fruit, so your life will be fruitless unless you live your life intimately joined to Mine."

How can you be intimately joined to Jesus? What would it look like if you were? What would have to change?

Romans 12:1 MSG—"So here's what I want you to do, God helping you: Take your everyday, ordinary life—your sleeping, eating, going-to-work, and walking-around life—and place it before God as an offering."

What are some specific practical ways I can focus my life on God?

John 15:7-8 TPT—"But if you step into My life in union with Me and if My words live powerfully within you—then you can ask whatever you desire and it will be done. When your lives bear abundant fruit, you demonstrate you are My mature disciples who glorify My Father."

How can mature disciples ask whatever they desire and it will be done for them?

Galatians 5:22-23 NLT—"But the Holy Spirit produces this kind of fruit in our lives: love, joy, peace, patience, kindness, goodness, faithfulness, gentleness, and self-control. There is no law against these things!"

What specifically does "bearing fruit" look like or what should it look like in your life? Give examples.

CREATE AND ACT

There are a lot of questions for you to answer in this chapter. Using the "Read and Write" section, break into small groups and answer as many of these questions as possible. Study this individually. Star or circle questions which challenge you and bring them up in the discussion time.

Number slips of paper 1-21. Fold and put in a container. Mix up the papers and have the women each choose a number. One at a time, have the women read their question and answer it. If it doesn't relate to them, have them choose another to answer.

1. What are the barriers to loving others?

2. Why do we try to hide our feelings from others?

3. Why is being open and honest scary? Is it for you?

4. What does it do to relationships when you wait to become perfect, to lose weight or accomplish some goal before connecting with others?

5.   In what ways does your weight or other imperfections keep you from loving others?

6.   Why do people manufacture reasons to keep others at arm's length?

7.   In what ways do you put up emotional walls because you are afraid others don't really love you?

8.   How has guilt about your weight or other issues affected your relationships?

9.   How has guilt about your weight or other issues affected your ability to invest in the time and energy it takes to overcome these issues?

10.   Why do changes first have to happen on the inside before they can move to the outside?

11.   Why does sharing your wants and needs with others feel risky and what can you do about that?

12.   What does it take for real intimacy to occur?

13.   What emotional needs do you have that move you toward bonding with others? To bonding with Jesus?

14.   In what ways do you erect barriers that keep you from bonding with others? To bonding with Jesus?

15.   Why is it necessary to apologize for your failures to those you are in close relationship with? When you know you have failed Jesus, do you apologize to Him and get His forgiveness? Why is this necessary? What happens if you don't do this?

16.   How can you be vulnerable with others? Why should you do this? How is it risky? Can you both guard yourself and be open? Think about how this would work in your life?

17. Do you have someone with whom you can be totally open? If you are married, are you open with your husband? Why or why not? What are you hiding or keeping back? How can you move towards being more open?

18. How is trust of those you are closest to relate to how you do or do not trust Jesus?

19. How do obedience, trust and intimacy go together in the Christian life?

20. Teresa says, "Each day I long to know Jesus more. So each day, I must trust Him more." How do we do this? Give specific examples.

21. Do you really trust Jesus? Do you trust Him with your physical health, your career, your finances? How about the safety and well being of your children, husband and/or parents?

EXCHANGES

Leaders: Hand out small pieces of paper or notecards to each participant.

On each card write an area you need to work on regarding the information in this chapter. It might be deepening trust, being open and vulnerable, practicing grace, apologizing, sharing how you feel or something you need to do in order to create a closer relationship with a specific person or with Jesus.

After writing these on the card, symbolically hand each area to Jesus and ask Him, what do you give me in exchange? Write what He gives you on the other side of the card or paper.

Then cross out the thing you gave Him . (Review Exchanges in the Principles section for more help.)

This is a process and it probably won't happen in one day. Make this a part of your everyday journey working to get close to Jesus and those around you. You can't live life alone, nor should you.

Spend some time sharing with a partner the areas you feel you need deeper emotional healing or areas God is working on healing.

PRAY AND SHARE

Leaders: Tell the members to spread out around the room and soak in God's presence as you play Kari Jobe's "The More I Seek You". Ask them to pray the prayer below and listento anything God says to them. Whatever He says, ask them to write it in their journal.

"Dear Jesus, thank You for healing my heart. Thank You for breaking down the walls that were keeping me from loving others and feeling love. I am worthy of love because You created me. Please help me continue to grow closer to You everyday. I seek true intimacy with You and with those closest to me. How can I step into life-union with You? In what ways can I make sure You are always at the center of my life? What areas do You need me to work on? Show me any areas that are holding me back from totally trusting You or others. I love You, Jesus. Help me to love You more."

Leaders: After the song, ask the members to rejoin you. Have cards you have prepared in advance. Use note cards without verses inside or blank heavy paper folded. You can decorate the outside if you wish. Inside each card, write one word.

All cards should be different meaningful words from scripture. Love, Joy, Peace, Patience, Goodness, Kindness, Self-Control, Faithfulness, Gentleness, Mercy, Grace, Truth, Power, Strength, Stand, Kneel, Courage, Encourage, Wisdom, Perseverance, Prosperity, Health, Discernment, Servant, Write, Sing, Dance, Dream, Soar, Fly, Stay, Run. Whatever words God leads you to write. Pray over each card as you prepare them asking God to deliver it to the right person. You will be giving these to the members, but you or they won't know what they are choosing.

Say: Remember I asked you at the beginning what was one thing you'd like to leave in this room tonight? You've probably done some things with that already. Let's do one final thing. I've prepared cards and have prayed over these. Each one has a word on them. I have this crazy faith. I believe God will allow you to choose the one word you need to help you deal with the issue you want to discard.

So right now, silently say to God, I give you whatever that one thing was. As I pass the basket, choose a card. It will contain a word that God is giving you to go forward. As the song plays ask God how you can use the power of that word to help you with the one thing you wanted to discard tonight. I'm going to play Kari one more time and I'll pass the basket. Mix up the cards and have the members choose one without looking. Play Kari Jobe's The Healer or another song as the basket is passed.

After everyone has gotten their words. Ask if anyone would like to share. Close in prayer.

FORGIVENESS

THINK ABOUT IT

Do you want God more than a cookie? Is there an area of your life that you would choose over God? (This would be like the rich young ruler choosing money.)

If so, this is your area of sin. Teresa admits one of her main areas of sin was eating foods made with sugar and flour. What is yours?

Do you love your sin more than God or are you willing to give this to God so He can give you something much greater?

Do you need God or do you feel there are some areas you can handle on your own?

Do you believe God's grace is enough to overcome your past sin and let you move on to the life He is calling you to lead?

If you jump in faith do you trust that God will catch you? In your mind, what does that look like?

READ AND WRITE

2 Cor. 12:9 MSG—"My grace is enough. It's all you need. My strength is made complete in your weakness."

How do grace and power work together in your life? How can you stand in His grace-power?

Philippians 4:11-13 TPT— "I know what it means to lack and I know what it means to experience overwhelming abundance for I'm trained in the secret of overcoming all things, whether in fullness or hunger. I find that the strength of Christ's explosive power infuses me to conquer any difficulty."

Have you experienced both lack and abundance, fullness and hunger? What are the difficulties with each of these? How can Christ's explosive power help you to overcome both?

1 Thessalonians 5:23 NIV—"May God Himself, the God of peace, sanctify you through and through. May your whole spirit, soul and body be kept blameless until the coming of our Lord Jesus Christ. The one who calls you is faithful, and He will do it."

What has God called you to do? How can He present every part of you blameless if you are holding part of you back? How will "He do it" as this Scripture says?

WHOLENESS WHEEL EXERCISE

Draw a circle and divide it into three pie sections. Label them body, soul, and spirit. Draw a scale on each line. Label the center point 0, and the edge of the circle 10. (Sample chart included.)

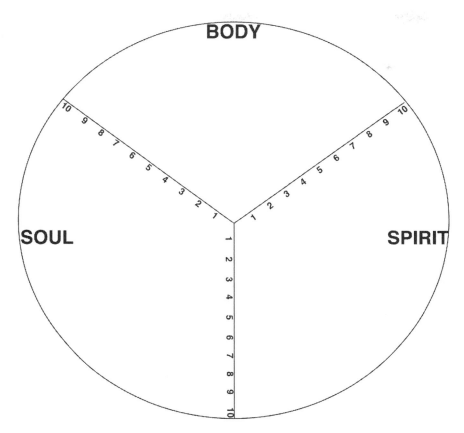

Rate yourself on these areas of your life. Remember your soul includes your mind, will and emotions so average how well you feel you're doing in all of those areas to get your score for your soul. The closer you are to the center, means the more work you still need to do. (Do you have a 10 body or a 1? Hey, you're at least a 1 because you are alive.)

What areas of your life are out of balance? Be specific about what in that area you feel is out of balance. For instance if it's your soul, note in your chart what area of your soul is out of balance? Do the same with spirit and body.

Now, color in the sections of your wheel to see how in balance your wheel is. Will it roll? Would it get you somewhere if you have four wheels like that on your car?

How can you get yourself in balance?

We have the power of God, Jesus, and the Holy Spirit to help move us towards wholeness. Hand your wheel to God. Ask Him what should I do first to get this wheel more in line with how You want me to be? Write down what He shows you. This is the beginning of your healthy living action plan.

SEA OF FORGETFULNESS EXERCISE

Ephesians 1:7-8 GW—"Through the blood of his Son, we are set free from our sins. God forgives our failures because of his overflowing kindness. He poured out his kindness by giving us every kind of wisdom and insight."

Do you keep a mental list of your sins? In your notebook, begin writing these down. Add to this list any ways you have caused others distress, inconvenience or harm because of your addictions, self-indulgences, weight, difficulties, despair or illnesses. Be sure to write down everything you can think of. We are going to ask God to throw these sins, worries and disappointments into the sea of forgetfulness.

Now using pens and paper provided by your leader, lightly write one word to sum up all that you have written. Turn these face down, don't crease or bend. We will do something with them in a minute. (Leaders, see note at the bottom of this section.)

Leaders: Purchase enough fingernail polish remover to soak all the papers for the entire group. For a large group this will be several large bottles of finger nail polish remover. More is better. Make sure it has no scents or dyes. Pour the fingernail polish remover in a small portable tub.

Those doing personal study can also try this exercise.

Micah 7:19 GW—"You will again have compassion on us. You will overcome our wrongdoing. You will throw all our sins into the deep sea."

Our Heavenly Father does not remember our sins. He throws them into the sea of forgetfulness and they are washed away. Today, we are going to do symbolically lay these sins on the altar and allow Him to take them from us. As we play some music, I want each of you to ask God to forgive you for the things you wrote on your paper. Then, taking the paper that symbolizes all your sins, as you feel led, take your paper to the tub, turn it face down and leave it. God is going to make these things disappear. He will remember them no more. We will revisit this sea of forgetfulness after a while.

Play "I Surrender" by Hillsong Live and/or "Altar" by Steve Fee. ("Altar" is available only on iTunes, Either of these are great songs for this activity. Personally, I prefer "Altar".)

BLOTTING OUT OUR SINS

The Sea of Forgetfulness is a fun activity. However, don't stress if you can't make it work An alternative activity is to write the main word on a piece of paper and then provide wide black permanent markers for them to blot out their sin by writing over it to the point they can no longer see it.

Mention these scriptures before you do the activity. Provide wide black markers so everyone can blot out their own difficulties.

Isaiah 43:25 NIV—"I, even I am He who blots out your transgressions, for my sake, and remembers your sins no more."

Acts 3:19 NKJV—"Repent therefore and be converted, that your sins may be blotted out, so that times of refreshing may come from the presence of the Lord."

PERSONAL NOTE FROM TERESA

I want everyone taking this course to know that the following Scriptures are my prayer for each of you, whether you are doing this study on your own or as a group. Groups, I know your leaders are also praying this for you. Listen as your leader reads this to you. Know that it comes from her heart. It certainly comes from mine. I love you and am praying for you to experience a level of sweet freedom that goes deeper than you ever dreamed possible.

PRAY, SHARE AND SING

Leaders, read the following prayer to the group.

Ephesians 1:16-21 NIV—"I have not stopped thanking God for you. I pray for you constantly, asking God, the glorious Father of our Lord Jesus Christ to give you spiritual wisdom and insight so that you may grow in your knowledge of God. I pray that your hearts will be flooded with light so that you can understand the confident hope He has given to those He called—His holy people who are His rich and glorious inheritance."

"I also pray that you will understand the incredible greatness of God's power for us who believe him. This is the same mighty power that raised Christ from the dead and seated him in the place of honor at God's right hand in the heavenly realms. Now He is far above any ruler or authority or power or leader or anything else—not only in this world, but also in the world to come."

Repeat the following affirmation out loud as a group or individual so that Satan hears from your own mouth whose you are!

"I am a child of the one true God. I can't live life on my own. I can't overcome temptation on my own, but I don't have to because I have the power of Jesus to lead me and protect me. He will keep my life balanced and on track if I turn over my life to Him. I willingly give You my life, Jesus. It is Yours. What do You give me in exchange?"

Listen carefully. As He gives you a gift, just shout it out for all to hear. Now, go to the sea of forgetfulness and get a visible glimpse of the fact that your sins are gone.

Song: Celebrate by playing "Our God" by Chris Tomlin. Crank it up. Sing along!

IMPORTANT NOTE TO LEADERS

If using The Sea of Forgetfulness activity, practice at home to make sure the type of paper, pens and fingernail polish remover do the work. Cut the paper into small squares. They are only to write one word to summarize their entire list. Cheap typing paper, which has NOT been run through a printer, works best. Make sure the paper you provide is identical to what you practiced on.

Black ink works best and stress writing lightly on the paper. You must have ink pens, not gel ink. Make sure you have the right kind of pens and each person writes with that pen on the type of paper you tested.

If you have a large group, purchase several large bottles of finger nail polish remover. The ink on the paper should dissolve in about five minutes. Before having the women come to the tank to see, check to make sure there are no legible words on any papers. We only want Jesus to have seen our sins!

THE PLACE THAT GRACE BUILT

THINK ABOUT IT

Do you feel like you are captive?

What put you in a captive circumstance?

What was the key to get you out of prison?

When did you get that key?

Why did you stay in prison if you had the key?

Why were you angry if you already had the key to get out?

Once you used the key to get free what or who kept calling you back?

How were you able to keep going toward freedom despite the perils?

What is the turning point in your journey towards freedom?

What keeps you going on your journey towards freedom?

What are some things you thought you wanted, but only enslaved you?

What does it mean to take up the thing, which is your biggest difficulty, and make it your greatest mission?

What does it mean to taste heaven?

What or where is the place that grace built?

READ AND WRITE

Luke 9:23 NIV—"Then he said to them all: 'Whoever wants to be my disciple must deny themselves and take up their cross daily and follow me.'"

What does it mean to deny yourself? What does that mean to you specifically?

What does it look like to you to take up your cross daily?

What does denying yourself have to do with following Jesus?

CREATE AND ACT

Create a reader's theater. Place the chairs in a semi-circle. Using the poem on pages 176-180, "The Place That Grace Built" choose people to read the stanzas out loud. Have enough study guides for each reader. Have the readers stand in front of the group in order of the stanzas they will read. Or if you have a person in the group who is a dramatic reader have them read the entire poem. Give the members several minutes to read over their parts. Give instructions to read their section as soon as the person ahead of them finishes.

Make this a creative time. Read the lines with appropriate expressions of anguish, tiredness, frustration, excitement, sadness, joy and elation.

If you are doing the study by yourself, read the poem out loud. Give emphases as you feel the words connecting to your spirit.

Don't worry if you cry. Tears wash the soul. Teresa always cries when she reads this poem out loud, so she will be disappointed if someone doesn't cry!

PRAY AND SHARE

John 8:36 NKJV—"Therefore if the Son makes you free, you shall be free indeed."

Share how the poem made you feel. Did you notice anything in the poem you hadn't seen before? What choices have you made on this journey? How has the Son set you free? What does it mean to be free indeed? How can you stay that way?

SING

Song: Play "Amazing Grace (My Chains are Gone)" by Chris Tomlin. Sing together.

Close by standing in a circle and having large group prayer. Allow the women to pray, as they feel led, having one person open and then have the leader close.

Leaders: Be available after this powerful session to share and pray with any who need to talk.

The Place That Grace Built

By Teresa Shields Parker

1. Shades of blacks and whites.
Long, black, angry shadows
Hiding fears, mistrusts and shame
And white as far as the eye can see.
Nothingness.
I wear my despair in monotone.
No cure for my sickness.
No help to pull me out of lifelessness.
No desire to climb to freedom.
Prison stripes. Prison bars.
Prison chains.
I am captive to myself.
I want to be free.
I want Someone to rescue me.
Unlock this bitter agony.
Set me free.

2. Silence is deafening.
I want to hear.
I demand to hear.
I know Someone is listening,
But no one answers.
Anger builds. Rage swells.
A fist raised to the sky.
Guttural anguish.
I want You to fix this.
I want to be loosed.
I demand an answer.
Ripping the stripes.
Pounding the bars.
Tugging at the chains.
It has to be easier than this.
How do I fix this?

3. A faint jingling
Could it be keys?
Could it be Someone is coming?
Could it be I will be set free?
He stops. He looks.
He weeps.
He turns to walk away.
Wait, don't leave.
Wait, You have the keys.
Wait, let me out.
His eyes bore into my soul.
Water and Fire,
Earth and Sky,
Birth and Death.
"My child, these keys are not yours.
You already have your key."

4. As quickly as He came, He left.
Though the words seemed a riddle
I remembered.
I knew the time.
I fell to my face.
I sobbed tears of regret.
I have lived my life for my own pleasures
And they have bound me.
I dressed myself in prison attire
And turned the lock myself.
I turned my back on His answers
Though He told me time and time again,
Surrender.
Repent.
Turn around.
Walk toward freedom.

5. Long, dark hallway.
Filled with perils
Leering from every corner,
Descending from every high place,
Grabbing hold and hanging on.
No, go away!
I am a child of obedience!
I am a child of freedom!
You will not capture me again!
Inch by inch. Step by step.
Choice by choice.
I am aware of a Power
Urging me forward,
The Wind at my back
Moving me closer to release,
Closer to the light of day.

6. Suddenly, there are colors,
Reds and pinks, Purples and blues,
Yellows and oranges,
The deep lush greens,
The brilliant hues of sunrise,
The dark browns of trees,
The grey-blue color of my lover's eyes,
The bright laughter of my daughter,
The slow smile of my son.
Feelings return and I embrace them.
I no longer push them away
For the drabness of my cell
Is something I will never forget.
I know what put me there.
I know what will keep me out.
I never want to go back.

7. What I thought I wanted
Only bound me tighter.
What I said I wanted
Seemed too hard
To fight for.
I tried, I tried to get free.
Beat my head against the wall.
Screamed at the top of my lungs.
Tried short-term fixes.
In the end,
He knew I had the key.
I knew I had the key.
I just didn't want to go through the pain
Of leaving the familiarity of my prison.
I had become comfortable there
In the place of death.

8. The light of day
Seemed so far out of reach.
I could never go there.
Only beautiful people live in color
And yet the Creator made me in color.
He created me for better things than prison,
But if I choose prison
He will allow me to stay there.
Choosing freedom
Is akin to choosing Him.
Though I did that long ago
I didn't know what it really meant
To deny myself
To take up the thing that is my biggest difficulty
And make it my greatest mission.
To follow and obey.

9. Now, I know.
Nothing tastes as good
As freedom feels.
Those sugary chains
Look delectable, taste like heaven,
But they hogtie like hell.
I've been to hell.
I never want to go back again.
I've tasted heaven.
I want to do whatever it takes
To stay close to the One who
Inhabits this glorious place.
This is the place that Grace built,
A place of safety, security,
Beauty, love, power.
I live here now.

L E S S O N   2 1

FINAL NOTE

THINK ABOUT IT

What battles have you faced?

How have you allowed the evil one to be the master puppeteer of your life?

How has your life changed after going on this journey?

What areas of your life have you given control to God?

What areas of your life do you still need to surrender?

How have you experienced Sweet Freedom?

READ AND WRITE

2 Chronicles 20:15 TLB—"The Lord says, 'Don't be afraid! Don't be paralyzed by this mighty army! For the battle is not yours, but God's!"

God is not saying in this Scripture that we don't do anything. Notice He tells Jehoshaphat to not be paralyzed by the enemy. Read the rest of this passage, from verses 16-30 and notice what happened.

With all that in mind, how can you allow God to fight your battles for you? How can you as a group help each other win your personal battles?

Ephesians 3:20 TPT—"Never doubt God's mighty power to work in you and accomplish all this. He will achieve infinitely more than your greatest request, your most unbelievable dream, and exceed your wildest imagination. He will outdo them all for His miraculous power constantly energizes you."

What does this tell us we should do instead of trying to makeup for all our shortcomings and failures? What weapon do we have at our disposal? How do we get this weapon?

What attributes of God do you relate to most? Find Scriptures, which proclaim these. See pages 238-239 in Sweet Freedom for some ideas.

CREATE AND ACT

Create a personal action plan for your healthy living journey. This may include things you are already doing. It should summarize what you have learned through this study.

I will include my responses so you see what kinds of things I want you to answer.

Don't use mine, though. You are a unique, child of God. He has a personal action plan just for you. Start where you are with what you know He's calling you to do.

Who are you and what do you want?

Example: I am a whole, healthy, happy woman who wants to fulfill the destiny God has for me.

What do you want God to do for you?

I desire for God's grace and the miraculous power of Jesus and the strength of the Holy Spirit to lead me always and remind me when I go astray.

How will you handle your emotions?

I ask that You, God, prompt me to recognize when an emotion is becoming how I am led. I promise to hand these debilitating emotions to You and ask, "What do you give me in exchange?" Then, I will accept those gifts and utilize them to fight the lies of the evil one. I promise to always go to You in times of hardship and struggle instead of being led by my emotions to food or other comforts I have run to in the past. I promise to forgive others whom I perceive have harmed me, to renounce the lies present in what I have believed about You and always ask for Your truth. I promise to be led by truth and the Word of God rather than what Imy emotions tell me I want in the moment.

How do you see yourself?

I will see myself through God's eyes. I will see that my failures can be great teachers and I determine they will not stop me from living my best life each and every day, holding tight to Jesus. I will see my small steps forward as part of the greater journey which leads me ever closer to my God.

How will you live from this day forward?

As a whole, healthy, happy woman I will concentrate on eating to fuel my body rather than my emotions. I will incorporate times of intentionally moving my body so it will become healthier. I will begin to embrace my emotions and seek to understand what they are showing me about myself rather than letting them lead my life. I will allow God to produce the fruit of the Spirit in my life, especially that of self-control. I will find coaches, mentors and fellow journeyers to connect with and help lead me forward to total health. Most of all, I will see feeding my spirit and focusing on following after God's Spirit as my number one goal in life.

What is your life mission?

I am a whole, healthy, happy woman administering grace and truth in a powerful way. I seek to allow Him to work in my life so I can fulfill the destiny He has for me.

What is a verse that describes your life mission?

"I am God's poetry, a recreated person who will fulfill the destiny He has given me, for I am joined to Jesus the Anointed One. Even before I was born, He planned in advance my destiny and the good works I would do to fulfill it." Ephesians 2:10 TPT (Personalized)

Save your answers in your journal. Type or write out on a separate piece of paper your full name and address and the answers to the last two questions. Bring this piece of paper to the last service. If this is that session, do that now.

COMMISSIONING SERVICE

Collect all the answers to the last two questions. Be sure each woman has her name and address on the sheet. For this service, a candlelight or low lighting atmosphere would be best. Prior to the service, make graduation certificates and print them out.

Note to Leaders: Each person does not have to have been at every meeting. If they consider themselves part of the group feel free to give them a certificate to encourage their continued journey.

It should have something like this on the certificate. Make it plain or fancy. Just make it up and print it on a computer.

This is to certify that

_____

(Name)

has completed the

Sweet Freedom Study

Held at

_____

(Location or Church Name)

On

_____

Dates

_____

Leader Signature

Leaders: Stand where everyone can see and hear you. Share a bit about what this group has meant to you and encouragement for continuing the journey. Mention Teresa has many different resources on her website and to be sure to connect with her in all the various ways in the book. Especially encourage them to subscribe to her website for updates and like her Facebook page.

Tell the members how proud you are of each one and how much it has meant to you personally that they have stayed with the journey.

Next read each member's Mission Statement and Mission Scripture. Call her to the front, say a few words, hand her the certificate and give her a hug. Invite the women those who want to gather round and pray short prayers for her. Tell them you will close. Do this for each woman.

SING

Song: Play "Clean" by Natalie Grant. Be sure to print out the lyrics for each participant. This was Teresa's inspiration song while writing *Sweet Freedom* and *Sweet Freedom Study Guide*. Stand in a circle and sing this closing song.

Give liberal hugs! And receive a virtual one from Teresa. She's sending them your way!

TO THE LEADERS

Two weeks after the study, mail each woman's mission statement page back to them with a personal note. By the way, leaders thanks for taking time to lead these meetings. It's hard to find dedicated leaders to take on these tasks. If I had a hat, I'd take it off and lay it at your feet. You are amazing.

A MESSAGE FROM TERESA

It's awesome having you ride along on this journey. I really would love it if you send me a note telling me how many members you had for your study. I'd love to hear any stories you want to tell me about your study times.

Did any breakthroughs happen?

What was your favorite session?

Were there sessions that just didn't work for you or your group?

What did you learn that knocked your socks off?

Did any members lose weight during your session. I mean it can be a long study if you do every lesson as a group.

If you did this study on your own, please send me an email about your experience as well.

Send all correspondence to Teresa@TeresaShieldsParker.com or info@TeresaShieldsParker.com.

FREE STUFF

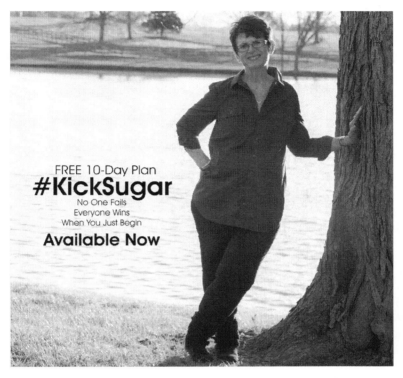

FREE 10-Day Plan
#KickSugar
No One Fails
Everyone Wins
When You Just Begin

Available Now

The 10-Video Course #KickSugar is FREE, and joining is simple and easy. Just go to TeresaShieldsParker. com. Click on the FREE tab and then on #KickSugar to begin your journey.

Under the FREE tab you'll find *Self-Sufficient*, the chapter she left out of *Sweet Freedom*. There are also selected chapters from *Sweet Grace* and *Sweet Change* under the FREE tab. There's even an ebook for aspiring writers: *How To Navigate Amazon and Launch Your Book*. It's all FREE. More gifts are added all the time.

TeresaShieldsParker.com

SELF-SUFFICIENT

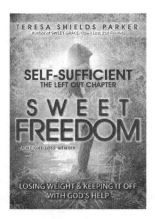

How does self-sufficiency sidetrack you on your weight loss? In your finances? In your ministry?

Teresa learned the answers to those questions and more. She shares her journey into self-suffiiency and out to His sufficiency. What she shares will help lead you to your own sweet freedom from feeling the crushing weight of having to bear the burden of doing it all yourself.

Self-Sufficient is probably the best *Sweet Freedom* chapter, but it's the one Teresa left out of the book. It stands alone and, therefore, she decided to offer it FREE to give a taste of what *Sweet Freedom* is all about. It's her gift when you subscribe to her website. Click on the FREE tab at TeresaShieldsParker.com and download it today!

WRITE A REVIEW

Please go to *Sweet Freedom* and *Sweet Freedom Study Guide* pages on Amazon and post reviews. With millions of books available any review long or short helps others discover *Sweet Freedom*. Teresa reads each one!

SWEET GRACE

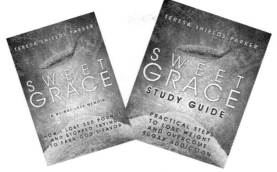

Sweet Grace: How I Lost 250 Pounds and Stopped Trying To Earn God's Favor is the #1 Christian weight loss memoir on Amazon. Teresa chronicles her journey of walking out of sugar addiction by the grace and power of God. She shares honestly and transparently about what it is like to be super morbidly obese, and what it takes to turn around and be free. Get your copy in print, kindle or audiobook on Amazon. Add *Sweet Grace Study Guide: Practical Steps To Lose Weight And Overcome Sugar Addiction* to use in conjunction with *Sweet Grace* for personal or group study.

"Excellent, lovingly written. Brings hope, encouragement and insight. Highly recommend." —Barb Thompson

"Thank you for being vulnerable and allowing the light of God to shine into your darkest places that we might see into ours. Love, love, love the chapter on grace!" —Luci Nicholson

"This is the most inspiring weight loss story I've ever read! This compelling story of God's grace is a must read for anyone struggling with food addiction. I saw myself on every page and believe I have found both the physical and spiritual answer to my own struggle." —Glenda Garcia

"Life-changing inspiration for the person who has been unable to understand the life long battle with food. End the yo-yo dieting and grasp the truth of this book." —Penney Anderson

SWEET CHANGE

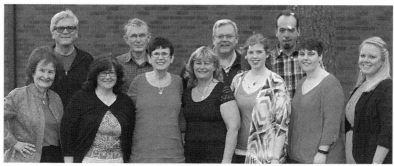

Teresa, center, with some of those featured in Sweet Change book.

Sweet Change: True Stories of Transformation is all about the power of change and how to tap into it. Teresa shares stories of individuals who have found their own personal ingredients work great with God's power in order to lose weight and step into transformation. Get your copy on Amazon today.

"This book is amazing! On vacation in Mexico I couldn't put it down. Thank you Teresa for this wonderful and inspiring book of Sweet Change." —Marjorie Eldredge

"Teresa Parker has done it again. Her first book Sweet Grace opened my eyes to my own sugar addiction. Sweet Change is filled with real life stories of men and women who have come to that moment of realization in their own lives, and made those steps towards changing bad habits and ultimately improving their health." —Anastacia Maness

"True stories of true transformation. The kind that only God can bring through a willing vessel. Thank you Teresa for another inspirational book for those of us on a life-long journey of weight loss transformation." —C. Turner

"This book will inspire and motivate anyone to change their life for the better." —Lindsey Summers

COACHING

Want Teresa's to help lead you to your transformation? Sweet Change Christian Weight Loss Coaching Group is for you. You'll receive support, encouragement, weekly videos, action steps, accountability, monthly live call, interaction with Teresa, 24/7 group access — all from a God-centered approach to weight loss. It's time for you to become free and healthy — body, soul and spirit.

Go to TeresaShieldsParker.com/Sweet-Change/

"Sweet Change group has given me a place to stop spinning in the midst of angst about needing to lose weight. I am gaining confidence I can change with God's help." —Carlene Coolley

"Sweet Change Group and the journey with Teresa Shields Parker is amazing and inspiring. Teresa's support, God's grace and the support of the group makes you stronger and reinforces your convictions." —Donna Barr

"I need a coach for direction and suggestions that work. I need the group to give and receive support. I need accountability and I love the spiritual support. I've lost 60 pounds and am nearly at my goal!" —Rhonda Burrows

"This has been exactly what I have needed to push through and continue on my journey."
—Heather Tucker

"Sweet Change awakened me to my special situation, and just kicking sugar for a few months resulted in a plateau-shattering 14-pound weight loss."
—Sharon Mello

#KICKWEIGHT

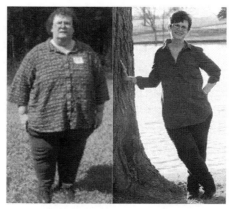

#KickWeight is Teresa's new low-cost, six-month coaching class. It is six months of learning the essentials of God-centered weight loss. This is not a diet and Teresa will give you a plan to follow. She will teach you how to develop your own healthy lifestyle plan, the one you will stay on for the rest of your life.

NO ONE-SIZE FITS ALL PLAN

Contrary to popular opinion, there is no one-size fits all weight loss plan. There are, however, some keys to figure out what works for you.

"#KickWeight is the place I suggest all my coaching clients begin," Teresa says. "We cannot start unless we know the basics. We've been told by every weight loss program, pill, shake or plan that theirs is the best. Let's allow God to lead us to His best plan for us."

As a coaching class, there will be a video with study guides and action steps every two weeks. For more information, to join (if the group is open) or to get your name on the wait list, go to TeresaShieldsParker.com/KickWeight/. Watch for information about new coaching classes!

IT'S HARD TO SAY GOOD-BYE!

PLEASE STAY CONNECTED

SUBSCRIBE to Teresa's website at TeresaShieldsParker.com for ongoing blog posts and updates on new books, products and free stuff!

FACEBOOK: www.facebook.com/TeresaShieldsParker.

TWITTER: Twitter.com/TreeParker.

PINTEREST: Pinterest.com/TreeParker.

INSTAGRAM: Instagram.com/TreeParker.

POST REVIEWS ON AMAZON REVIEWS on any and all of her books.

INVITE TERESA TO SPEAK at your group, church, Bible study, small group, Women's club, health fair or event.

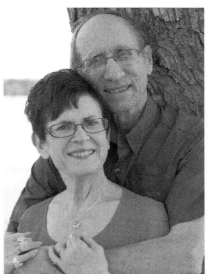

HOST a *Sweet Grace* or *Sweet Freedom* study group in your community, church or club, and let us know about it.

EMAIL your questions to info@TeresaShieldsParker.com.

Teresa and Roy Parker

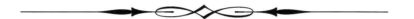

"We have become His poetry, a recreated people that will fulfill the destiny He has given each of us, for we are joined to Jesus, the Anointed One. Even before we were born, God planned in advance our destiny and the good works we would do to fulfill it!"

Ephesians 2:10 TPT

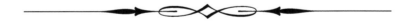

198

Made in the USA
San Bernardino, CA
05 December 2016